Medicine From The Heart

Matt —

I love you
with all my heart.
This book comes
from my heart
to yours

Dad

Medicine From The Heart

Bernard Leo Remakus, M.D.

Writers Club Press
San Jose New York Lincoln Shanghai

Medicine From The Heart

Writers Club Press
an imprint of iUniverse, Inc.

For information address:
iUniverse, Inc.
5220 S. 16th St., Suite 200
Lincoln, NE 68512
www.iuniverse.com

ISBN: 0-595-24502-1

Printed in the United States of America

This book is dedicated to physicians—
past, present, and in the making.

Contents

INTRODUCTION

I published my first article in a medical journal in 1980. Since that time, I have contributed over 200 articles to the medical literature.

Some of these articles were research findings and some were clinical observations, but most were medical essays. Many of my essays have been reprinted in non-medical publications, while others have been used to help teach various courses in American medical colleges and universities.

Although most of my essays have been directed at a physician audience, they have been read by people from many different walks of life. Among my souvenirs are letters from presidents of the United States, congressmen, religious leaders, lawyers, businessmen, physicians, and other professionals, who took the time to personally thank me for different articles I have written.

In recent years, a number of physicians have requested that I publish a collection of essays in book form, as have other individuals who work outside the medical profession and have had limited access to my writing. In the past, publishing such a book always seemed like something I would do at a future date, but the precarious state of health care in the United States today, as well as the fragile state of the world at large, have made me realize that there could not be a more opportune time to share the message of hope.

MEDICINE FROM THE HEART is a collection of 50 essays that deal with the human side of medicine. Each essay tells a different story about some very special people, some very important events in their lives, and how these events have been shaped by the on-going metamorphosis of America's health care delivery system.

My patients, colleagues, and family are the substrate from which each of these essays has been woven. Pertinent issues currently influencing American health care, as well as issues that have been debated by physicians from the earliest days of Medicine, provide the backdrop.

The stories conveyed in my essays are true stories about real people and real experiences. In some essays, the names have been changed either to protect the innocent or to facilitate the layout of this book.

The opinions conveyed in these essays are mine and mine alone. I do not expect every reader to agree with every word I have written, but I do expect every reader to consider each story within the framework of their own knowledge and experience, and in doing so, to formulate their own opinions and conclusions about the topics discussed herein.

I have always found it rewarding to have readers understand and accept my point of view. However, I have always found it much more rewarding to get people thinking about an issue, even when the process resulted in contrasting opinions or different conclusions.

For the past 22 years, I have practiced medicine in rural America. Unencumbered by the distractions of medicine as practiced in the big city, I have had the time to experience, reflect, and write.

The pages that follow convey my experiences and reflections. These pages tell the story of one man's attempt to practice medicine the only way he knew—from the heart.

August, 2002

MY TRAVELS WITH RAY

I had just finished admitting Ray to the hospital when my office phone rang.

"Can you tell me why this patient requires hospitalization?" the young woman asked, identifying herself as a representative of a major health insurer.

"Ray's no longer covered by your company," I replied, trying to be helpful. "He's on Medicare now."

"I know that," the secretary insisted. "We still need the information so that we can authorize his admission before we deny his benefits."

Too tired to engage in unnecessary dialogue or to try to understand the peculiar logic of the insurance industry, I decided to simply cooperate and tell the secretary about my 60 year-old patient.

"Ray has chronic obstructive pulmonary disease," I began, "as well as an advanced, inoperable narrowing of the trachea. He breathes through a plastic tube in his throat, but infected secretions are starting to fill the tube. He's on home oxygen, but he had a very difficult time breathing last night. This morning, he was weak, dehydrated, and febrile, and his white count was 17,000."

"Couldn't he be managed at home?" the secretary inquired.

"I don't think you get the picture," I replied with uncharacteristic patience. "Once upon a time, this man was accidentally thrown forward in a truck cab, and a gear shift went into his throat, crushing his trachea. Since that time, numerous surgical procedures have left him with a throat full of scar tissue. His last surgical procedure was experimental, and a small plastic tube is this man's only remaining airway. I have been taking care of him for the past 12 years, and I have developed a pretty healthy understanding of when I can treat him at home and when I have to admit him to the hospital."

"Does he have any other medical problems?" the secretary asked.

"A few," I replied, as I prepared to recite a litany of his active medical problems. "For starters, he has coronary vascular disease, congestive heart failure, hypertension, diabetes mellitus, peptic ulcer disease, cholelithiasis, herniated cervical discs, herniated lumbo-sacral discs, assorted radiculopathies, crippling osteoarthritis, symptomatic benign prostatic hypertrophy……"

"I see," the secretary interrupted. "Alright, we can approve him for 3 days."

"Don't you want to hear the rest of his diagnoses?" I asked. "I haven't even gotten to the good stuff yet."

"No, that will be fine. Thank you, Doctor," the secretary replied, quickly hanging up the phone.

Comforted by the fact that Ray's hospitalization was being approved for 3 days by a company that no longer insured him, I went about my usual business of giving Ray the best possible medical care. I also went about my usual business of refusing to allow the directives of health insurers interfere with the care of my patients.

For the first few days of his hospitalization, Ray appeared to be improving—but then the inevitable finally happened. Following years of suffering the cumulative effects of multiple incapacitating illnesses, Ray's heart could no longer take the strain.

Following Ray's death, I spent the entire morning at the hospital, comforting his wife, the majority of his 10 children and 22 grand-children, and a few close friends. A few days later, I delivered the eulogy at Ray's funeral.

While preparing Ray's eulogy, I relived many of the experiences we had shared in our 12-year association. Although I tried to concentrate on our happier moments together, I couldn't help but think about some of the sub-optimal experiences we had also shared.

I couldn't help but think about our many fights with hospital billing departments, insurance companies, Workmen's Compensation, the Disability bureau, and Medicare. Ray's insurance coverage was constantly being punted from one insurance company or federal agency to another, and the incessant phone calls and letters from his insurers discouraged Ray and made him feel like a burden.

I couldn't help but think about how laymen were always trying to dictate the length of Ray's hospital stays, and how no one ever seemed to understand the nature of his problems. A peer review organization even gave me a tough time once for treating Ray with intravenous hydrocortisone for a week and not placing him on oral prednisone at the time of discharge.

The reviewer didn't seem to care that Ray didn't need prednisone as an outpatient or that he had many contraindications to the chronic use of the drug. The reviewer seemed more concerned about keeping Ray out of the hospital, and he seemed to think that this could be achieved by placing Ray on chronic steroid therapy.

I couldn't help but think about the sacrifices Ray had to make just to be able to afford many of his medications. Ray lived just above the poverty line and didn't qualify for drug assistance.

On one occasion, Ray was told by another physician that "his doctor should learn about sustained-release theophylline preparations." Ray, who had long profited from aminophylline, which he took four times daily, didn't know how to tell the other physician that he couldn't afford the expensive sustained-release capsules.

He also didn't know how to tell the other physician that "his doctor" routinely bought his aminophylline and a number of other medications from a wholesale drug company without any charge to Ray and without any reimbursement from his insurers. Ray didn't know how to explain many things to many people who were only temporarily or peripherally involved in his complicated health care, so he swallowed his pride and generally offered very few explanations at all.

I couldn't help but think about the difficulty Ray had each time he was sent to a major referral center. Ray was just an extraordinarily-ill human being who only wanted the medical or surgical care he couldn't receive at a small rural hospital but, more often than not, he was seen as a malpractice suit waiting for a place to happen.

On one occasion, a compassionate otolaryngologist agreed to perform experimental surgery on Ray with the hope of reconstructing his diseased airway and sustaining his life. Feeling threatened by a potential malpractice suit, the otolaryngologist's partner refused to assist in the surgery.

To make matters worse, the otolaryngologist's partner, who wanted nothing to do with the case, even refused to order badly-needed medications for Ray post-operatively. Ray suffered an entire week-end in a hospital bed because of an arrogant physician's misconceptions.

Thinking about all our experiences together made me realize that I had walked with Ray down many different roads. It also made me realize that caring for Ray had forced me to take a close look at many of the things that were wrong with our health care delivery system.

Following Ray's funeral, each member of his family came up to me and thanked me for caring for their father. Their embraces, tears, and kind words were as sincere as any I have ever known.

"Thank you, Bernie," one of Ray's daughters said, hugging me. "We never would have had him this long without your help."

In the many years that I labored to preserve Ray's life, I became well aware of everything that was wrong with the practice of medicine. It took Ray's death to remind me of everything that was still right with it.

January, 1994

FAITH AS MEDICINE

O ne of the most beautiful and serene spots on this entire planet is the Grotto of Our Lady of Lourdes in Emmitsburg, Maryland. Ensconced in a lush and fragrant mountainside, the grotto overlooks the stately buildings of Mount Saint Mary's College, as well as the lavish farmlands that form the southern boundary of the Mason-Dixon Line.

The grotto is the site where Mother Elizabeth Seton once taught, and where water reputed to possess healing properties quietly runs past various altars and statues. It is the site where visitors have reported seeing the Blessed Mother and where more than an occasional miracle is said to have transpired.

If you ever visit the grotto, you will be overcome by its beauty, as well as the appearance of many of its visitors. Children with terminal illnesses, crippled adults in obvious pain, and young, infertile couples are just some of the many visitors who frequent the grotto to pray, partake of the spiritual waters, and wait for a miracle.

Most of the sick and dying who visit the grotto have previously seen many different health care providers in many different professional settings, but have been unable to obtain the treatment, cure, or relief they need. Most of these individuals visit the grotto to seek from faith, religion, and prayer that which they have been unable to obtain from the science of medicine.

The concept of religious faith as medicine is as old as mankind itself. Most civilizations that have promoted religious faith have also fostered the belief that God heals, and that faith and prayer can promote and restore health.

In recent decades, the medical literature has been reluctant to explore how religious faith seems to promote health and longevity in much the same way that contemporary American society has been reluctant to allow the concept of "one nation under God" to manifest itself in our public schools. In recent months, however, the medical literature has joined the rest of the news media in trying to explain the role of prayer and religion in the process of healing.

The October, 1999 edition of *Reader's Digest* featured an article entitled, *"Faith Is Powerful Medicine,"* which commented on more than 30 scientific studies that have found a connection between religious faith and health. A number of these studies concluded that church members had lower death rates than non-members regardless of risk factors such as smoking, drinking, obesity, and inactivity; that those with a religious commitment had better outcomes in 7 of 8 cancer studies, 4 of 5 blood pressure studies, 4 of 6 heart disease studies, and 4 of 5 general health studies; and that similar connections existed between religion and health in young children as well as older adults, in people who suffered from acute illnesses as well as those who suffered from chronic diseases, and in U.S. Protestants as well as European Catholics, Japanese Buddhists, and Israeli Jews.

The findings of these scientific studies are in line with the popular sentiment of patients and physicians alike. Recent *Time/CNN* and *USA Weekend* polls demonstrated that 80% of Americans believe that faith or prayer can help people recover from illness or injury, while 99% of physicians surveyed at a recent meeting of the American Academy of Family Physicians felt that religion contributed to healing.

There are a number of scientific theories that have attempted to explain how prayer heals. These include the hypotheses that religion guarantees social support which is a recognized key to health and longevity; that organized religion teaches people how to better handle illness, suffering, and loss; and that the physical act of praying leads to a lowering of blood pressure, decreases in metabolic, heart, and respiratory rates, the formation of a relaxation response, and a reduction in stress.

These theories, of course, fail to explain how prayer heals others. In a 1988 study by San Francisco cardiologist, Randolph Byrd, nearly 400 heart patients were divided into two groups, with only one group receiving the prayers of volunteers from all over America.

The study concluded that patients in the group receiving prayers experienced fewer complications, fewer cases of pneumonia, fewer cardiac arrests, fewer bouts of congestive heart failure, and required fewer antibiotics than patients in the group that did not receive prayers. Significantly, patients in this study did not know to which group they had been assigned.

Scientific theories notwithstanding, could prayer heal because there really is a God who answers prayers and who has the capacity to heal? Similarly, could religious faith be connected to health and longevity because people of faith are willing to accept illness and suffering as temporary and manageable phenomena, trust in God's ability to intercede and protect, and view their current existence as only one step in the continuum of eternal life?

Regardless of your own religious beliefs, it is incontrovertible that a definite relationship between religious faith and health exists, as does the potential for faith to serve as powerful medicine. Any study that attempts to link religious belief and physical well-being can be explained scientifically or criticized on the basis of experimental design, but what cannot be explained or denied as easily are the numerous instances in which patients unexpectedly overcame profound illness and credited their survival to God's intervention.

As physicians, it would be inappropriate to impose our own religious beliefs on patients in the clinical setting. However, it would be just as inappropriate to disregard the religious beliefs of our patients or exclude faith, religion, or prayer from the healing process.

Faith is powerful medicine. It should be embraced as a highly effective therapeutic modality, and its use encouraged in the healing process of religious patients and their families.

When asked in the movie, ***Oh, God,*** if Jesus was his son, God, as portrayed by George Burns, answered, "Yes, Jesus is my son, and so is Buddha, and so is Moses." As physicians, we should welcome the opportunity to embrace faith in each of its many forms.

Whenever I visit the Grotto of Our Lady of Lourdes, I say a quiet prayer for those who have come to the grotto searching for relief from their illness and suffering. I also say a prayer for the many dedicated physicians who have done everything humanly possible to help these patients.

During my professional lifetime, I have encountered a few physicians and patients who felt that the physician's office and the medical literature were not the proper places to discuss religion. During this same lifetime, I have met many more physicians and patients who have welcomed faith, religion, and prayer as intricate and inseparable parts of the healing process.

From an inscription on a pulpit at the Grotto of Our Lady of Lourdes, I have learned how to keep the matter of faith as medicine in the proper perspective. The inscription reads: "For those who believe in God, no explanation is necessary; for those who do not believe in God, no explanation is possible."

October, 1999

UNDERSTANDING THE HIPPOCRATIC OATH

A n oath is generally accepted as a ritualistic declaration of one's intent to speak the truth, keep a promise, or remain faithful. A prime example of such a declaration is the Hippocratic Oath which most of us took during our medical school graduation ceremonies as an expression of our willingness to perform ethically as physicians.

In recent years, a number of physicians have criticized the Hippocratic Oath as an impractical anachronism. However, the fact does remain that most physicians swore to uphold the tenets of the Oath as we prepared to embark on our careers in Medicine.

When each of us recited the Hippocratic Oath, we swore "...to reckon him who taught me this Art equally dear to me as my parents, to share my substance with him, and relieve his necessities if required; to look upon his offspring in the same footing as my own brothers, and to teach them this art, if they shall wish to learn it, without fee or stipulation..." In other words, we promised to respect and share our knowledge and good will with one another.

We also pledged to promote a sense of solidarity within our profession and develop ways of taking care of our own. At no time did any of us pledge to treat each other with arrogance, to speak of each other in denigrating terms, or to give unfavorable accounts of each other's work for the mere sake of personal profit, as frequently occurs in peer review and expert testimony.

When we took the Hippocratic Oath, we also pledged to "...follow that system of regimen which, according to my ability and judgment, I consider for the benefit of my patients…" In other words, we promised to make the health of our patients our most important priority.

At no time did any of us pledge to compromise the health and well-being of our patients so that we might stay in compliance with the payment guidelines of health insurers. At no time, did we pledge to abbreviate the care of our patients so that our HMO accounts might stay balanced.

With the words, "I will give no deadly medicine to any one if asked, nor suggest any such counsel; and in a like manner I will not give to a woman a pessary to produce abortions…," we swore that we would use our knowledge and ability to heal rather than kill. We swore that we would not market death machines or become employed as executioners, just as we swore that we would not assist in the termination of unborn life.

We never swore that we would not do everything in our power to help a dying patient achieve a peaceful and painless death, or that we would not rescue a woman whose life was threatened by the complications of pregnancy. We only swore to become instruments of life, rather than death, and to leave the termination of life to that greater power from which life originates.

By pledging, "Into whatever houses I enter, I will go into them for the benefit of the sick, and will abstain from every other voluntary act of mischief and corruption; and, further, from the seduction of females or males, of freemen and slaves…," we promised to maintain a certain sanctity in our relationship with patients. We also promised not to usurp any power we might attain as a result of our tenure in the medical profession.

We never promised to take advantage of the frailty of the human condition in any way, shape, or form. Similarly, we never promised to abuse our power within our profession or outside its boundaries.

In taking the Hippocratic Oath, we also pledged that, "Whatever, in connection with my professional practice or not, in connection with it, I see or hear, in the life of men, which ought not to be spoken of abroad, I will not divulge, as reckoning that all such should be kept secret..." In other words, we pledged to protect the confidentiality of our patients and our colleagues.

We never promised to profit personally in any way by divulging the shortcomings of other physicians. We never promised to compound the adversity of our patients by making their problems a matter of public record.

Many physicians look upon their recitation of the Hippocratic Oath with almost as much reverence as a polygamist looks upon his recitation of marriage vows. Such physicians view the Hippocratic Oath as a ceremonial appurtenance that was never meant to be taken literally.

Conversely, other physicians view the Hippocratic Oath as a bona fide code of professional conduct and an eloquent expression of timeless wisdom. These physicians continue to view Medicine as a calling rather than a mere profession, and seem to have little trouble claiming that, "...with purity and with holiness I will pass my life and practice my Art..."

Not that many years ago, most of us finished our one and only recitation of the Hippocratic Oath with the words, "While I continue to keep this Oath unviolated, may it be granted to me to enjoy life and the practice of the art, respected by all men, in all times! But should I trespass and violate this Oath, may the reverse be my lot!"

Although we may not have realized it at the time, our reading of the Hippocratic Oath may have provided Medicine with answers to some of its most pressing ethical questions. Maybe somebody is trying to tell us something.

January, 1992

PURPOSE

I n this ever-changing world, there are very few constants in any of our lives. I feel fortunate to have the unconditional love of my family as a constant in my own life.

I also feel fortunate to have a number of other constants. One of these constants is my yearly letter from Jerry.

I first met Jerry in the emergency room of a small rural hospital nine years ago. I remember him as being in his early fifties, markedly overweight, and a few ventricular fibrillations away from shuffling off this mortal coil.

Jerry had come to the Pennsylvania mountains for a summer respite from a stressful job in New Jersey. While chopping fire wood, he started to develop chest pain, and one massive myocardial infarction later, he was brought to our emergency room where he promptly had the first of his two cardiac arrests.

Following our first round of cardio-pulmonary resuscitation and advanced cardiac life support, Jerry was moved from the emergency room to the intensive care unit where he promptly had his second cardiac arrest. Following a second exhaustive resuscitative effort, it became apparent that Jerry had developed a third-degree atrio-ventricular block and his heart had lost its ability to function normally.

With little alternative, I hooked Jerry up to the hospital's only portable cardiac monitor and wheeled him into the hospital's Radiology Department, the site of the hospital's only fluoroscopy unit. There, with the aid of the ICU's only available nurse, I inserted the hospital's only temporary transvenous pacemaker, a nifty little unit that had been collecting dust on an ICU shelf longer than anyone seemed to remember.

Once the pacemaker had been inserted, I moved Jerry back to the ICU where I spent the better part of the following week handling his myocardial infarction, third-degree atrio-ventricular block, ventricular arrhythmia, congestive heart failure, cardiogenic shock, and pericarditis. Within two weeks, Jerry was totally asymptomatic and discharged from the hospital.

Shortly after Jerry had been chalked up in the "save" column, another physician, who was big on peer review, special committees, and physician investigations, started to make a fuss about the way I handled Jerry's case. This physician argued that Jerry should have been transferred by ambulance to a larger hospital forty minutes away immediately following his cardiac arrest in our emergency room.

The physician contended that small rural hospitals were not equipped to handle complicated medical cases. The fact that Jerry would have died en route to another hospital without the placement of a pacemaker and immediate intensive medical treatment was inconsequential to the disgruntled physician, as was the fact that Jerry and his wife had declined the option of transfer to a larger facility when his stabilization made such a transfer feasible.

Every defense of Jerry's treatment was inconsequential to this physician and her committee except the defense that was made by a renowned university cardiologist, who examined Jerry and his records and who had little trouble concurring with every aspect of Jerry's treatment. "I closely reviewed every word in your medical records," the cardiologist told Jerry, "and I firmly believe that, if your doctor had made any one of his many decisions differently, you would have never made it out of that hospital alive."

Every year, I get a card or letter from Jerry reminding me of how we met nine years ago. I just received this year's entry—a postcard from the Florida Keys, where Jerry and his wife are currently fishing.

As I read Jerry's note, I began to realize how fortunate I am to have a number of patients who routinely go out of their way to express their gratitude for my medical care. To be sure, there is no surplus of gratitude for what any of us does to maintain the health of our patients, but Jerry's note reminded me that there is some gratitude.

Jerry's note also reminded me of one of our profession's most intriguing paradoxes. It reminded me that, regardless of our competence or compassion, we must all repeatedly defend our every action and continually fight for the right to ease the pain and suffering of our fellow man.

As if myocardial infarctions and heart blocks were not enough to handle, physicians also have to contend with many groups of difficult individuals. They include the feds, the insurance companies, the malpractice lawyers, a medically-ignorant body of lawmakers, and those in the medical profession who still do not seem to understand their own true purpose.

A doctor's fundamental purpose is the care of his or her patients. Unfortunately, there are many forces in society that would divert the attention of physicians from such an obvious truism.

Each of us in Medicine owes our patients and our profession too much to ever allow these forces to obscure the nobleness of our purpose. Our patients and profession are our first and foremost responsibility.

The front of Jerry's most recent postcard is an aerial photograph of the Florida Keys. One of the Keys has been circled and a large arrow points to the hand-written message, "Because of you, I'm here."

No, Jerry, it's because of you that I'm here.

August, 1992

A BARE PATCH OF GROUND

Spring is a beautiful time of year in the rural mountains of North-eastern Pennsylvania. The sun returns from its winter vacation, the air becomes fragrant with honeysuckle and lilac, and the countryside starts to glow with a verdant hue.

By the time summer arrives, everything in and about this area turns into a lush shade of green. Well, almost everything.

On the 14 acres I call home, there is a bare patch of ground on which grass refuses to grow. This circular patch measures 5 feet in diameter and is prominent at one end of an otherwise green field of mixed grasses.

For many years, my wife has tried to fill in the bare patch with various combinations of grass seed and fertilizers, but all of her efforts have been for naught. Individual blades of grass have periodically appeared in the patch, but their stay has been short-lived.

Once upon a time, all kinds of grass grew in the patch—rye, red fescue, even Kentucky blue grass. But that was before my 16 year old son, Chris, started playing baseball.

For some reason, Chris chose that patch of ground for his batter's box—the place where he would learn to hit a baseball. Over the past decade, Chris has hit thousands of baseballs from that same spot, and with each new time at bat, each new movement of dirt with his spikes, and each new powerful swing, more and more grass has decided to leave the patch.

Chris just finished his sophomore year in high school, and during this past baseball season, he led his varsity team in nearly every hitting category. He was recently named to the high school All-Star team, and college baseball programs are already starting to recruit him.

Chris was the first to use that patch of ground as a batter's box, but it didn't take long for my other children to follow his lead. My 14 year-old daughter, Ali, and my 11 year-old son, Matt, also learned the art of hitting on that same spot.

For the past few years, Ali has been one of the top softball players in this part of the state. She will be playing in All-Star tournaments in a number of different states this summer, and it will be worth the drive just to watch the opposing outfielders back up to the fence every time she steps up to the plate.

During the same period of time, Matt has also become one of the stars of his little league. Like Ali, he will also be playing in All-Star tournaments this summer, and with each time at bat, he will be getting closer to breaking the hitting records Chris set when he was in the little league.

The hitting ability of my children is no accident. Having played baseball my entire life, I have learned a trick or two about hitting, and having coached the game at the high school level, I have learned how to teach the art.

For many years, I have been stepping on to that bare patch of ground and teaching my kids how to hit. In doing so, I have gotten to know more about my kids and more about myself.

Many years ago, the wife of an aging country doctor lamented that her husband never took the time to know his children and that his children were never given the opportunity to know him. The lesson stuck with me more than anything I ever learned in medical school.

The lesson was one of the reasons I moved to the country and one of the reasons I built a medical office in my home. My family has always been my highest priority, and with a little imagination, I have been able to enjoy all the benefits of a rich family life without having to sacrifice a busy medical practice, writing career, or assorted other avocations.

While my kids were taking batting practice today, I wondered what the future held for each of them. My two sons have mentioned professional baseball, and even my daughter has talked about playing baseball in a professional women's league that is now being formed.

My kids have also talked about a few other possible career choices, including Medicine and writing. Insofar as they have all been blessed with smarts and have solid academic credentials, it would appear that there is no limit to their list of possible careers.

A few months ago, the ***American Medical News*** ran an open letter from a physician to his son. In the letter, the physician tried to explain to his son why he could not attend concerts, coach little league, or do a lot of the other things that fathers, who did not have the time constraints or responsibilities of a physician, could do.

In his letter, the physician went on to explain the demands, politics, and current state of disarray of the medical profession. He concluded his letter by advising his son not to become a physician.

Only a physician could understand the rigors of medical school and residency, the effects of sleep deprivation, and the unglamorous substrate upon which medicine is practiced. Only a physician could understand the pressures of the malpractice epidemic, the constant hassle of Medicine's third party, and the uncertainty of health care reform.

Only a physician could understand what his or her life is and what it might have been in another profession. Only a physician could feel the kind of frustration that would prompt him to discourage his son from following in his footsteps.

I do not know if any of my children will ever dream of becoming a doctor, but if they do, I want them to be able to pursue that dream without any reservations. To this end, I feel obligated to do what I can to help restore our profession to its rightful place in society.

The medical profession currently has more than its fair share of problems, but our problems have very little to do with the practice of medicine. Our problems are political and socio-economic in nature,

and as such, are problems that our profession can solve with a concerted effort from all our members.

It is not my nature to hoist a white flag and give up my ground; it is
my nature to fight. Accordingly, I refuse to give in to the lawyers, legislators, and businessmen who are trying to take my profession away
from me.

I feel an obligation to protect the medical profession not just for my
children or the children of my medical colleagues, but also for all the
other children who were born with the dream of becoming a doctor. As
physicians, we have a responsibility, not only to our patients, but also
to our profession and to those who will serve and be served by our profession in years to come.

In the not-so-distant future, my children will all be pursuing their
own careers. If Medicine attracts any of them, I can only hope that
some of the problems currently plaguing the medical profession will
have been eliminated.

Being very close to my children, I share all their dreams and I do all
I can to help ensure their futures. In all honesty, however, I try not to
think about the day when they will have all moved away.

The backyard won't be the same without 3 kids playing baseball. It
won't be the same without that bare patch of ground.

July, 1994

THE ART OF MEDICINE

I first met Sara twenty years ago while I was helping her husband survive his first heart attack. During his hospitalization, I spoke with Sara on many separate occasions and learned that she was an artist.

Both Sara and her husband were very grateful for my medical care, and following her husband's hospitalization, she invited me to their home to select one of her paintings as a gift. Months passed, and despite endless calls and personal invitations to select a painting, I found myself too busy to drive five-minutes and select a work of art that I was sure would be of the "paint-by-numbers" genre.

One day, as I was visiting a local bank, I was amazed at the beautiful works of art that were being displayed by a local artist in the bank's lobby. To say that I was dumbfounded when I discovered that the paintings were the work of my patient, Sara, is a profound understatement.

A few days later, Sara came to my office with her husband and once again inquired when I would be stopping by their home to pick out my painting. "This afternoon," I replied enthusiastically, never indicating that I had seen her exhibit at the local bank.

When I arrived at Sara's home, I was amazed at the dozens of beautiful paintings that adorned her walls. "You can have any painting, but this one," Sara said to me, as she showed me her most famous painting—a perennial first-place winner at the county fairs of New York and Pennsylvania.

Although I carefully studied every painting in Sara's home, I kept returning to the one painting she told me I couldn't have. I was overwhelmed by the colors, shadowing, and details of the painting, and couldn't spend enough time studying it.

As I tried to understand how Sara had been able to paint half of a stone barn and field in a shadow and the other half in sunlight, the artist returned to the room and detected my obvious attraction for her special work of art. "Will you take that painting already and get out of here?" she chided.

"I wouldn't think of taking your prize painting," I replied, "but it's so beautiful, I can't take my eyes off it."

Taking the painting down from her wall, Sara took one last look at it and handed it to me. "I'll have you know that you are the only person alive who I would give this painting to," she said with obvious sincerity.

A few years later, her husband had his second heart attack, and following his hospitalization, I was once again invited to Sara's home to select a painting as a gift. Responding quickly, I visited her home and was immediately told that I could have any painting but that of a wooden chair upon which a potted plant had been placed and a filigreed shawl draped.

"I'd let you have that one, but I've already been commissioned to paint it for someone else," Sara said. Seeing my immediate attraction for the painting, she took it off the wall, handed it to me, and said, "Here, take it. The other person will just have to wait for me to paint it again!"

The walls of my office waiting room are adorned with five of Sara's paintings. Each of the paintings has a story, as do my other office paintings that have been given to me by other patients.

One of these paintings, a beautiful depiction of an old mill on a tranquil pond, was given to me by my patient, Ray. It was his daughter's first painting following her art studies, and a gift to her father.

"This is the only worldly possession I have that means anything to me," Ray said with tears in his eyes, as he presented the painting to me. "A gift only means something when it's all you have to give."

I call the collection of paintings in my office, "The Art of Medicine." There's not a day that goes by that I don't look at each of these paintings and recall the many wonderful memories associated with the patients who were responsible for placing the paintings on my previously unadorned walls.

Many years ago, I discovered that the formula for success as a physician could be stated in the equation, $S = A + A + A$. "S" stands for success, and the three "A's" are: availability, affability and ability.

I have practiced medicine in rural Northeastern Pennsylvania for more than two decades, and during that time, I have taken pride in always trying to be there when my patients needed me, treating my patients as I would my friends or family, and providing the best medical care possible. To this end, I have kept a 24/7 phone line open for my patients and encouraged them to use it when necessary, taken the time to know my patients as people first and patients second, and made every effort to stay current with my profession, provide affordable medical care, and actively fight any outside forces that would attempt to compromise the needs of my patients or the quality of my work.

Life has not always been easy as a rural physician, nor has it been lucrative to the point of promoting independence of wealth. What it has been is rewarding, fulfilling, and by most measures and observations, successful.

During my medical training, I was taught that Medicine is a science, but following more than two decades of private practice, I have come to the realization that Medicine is just as much an art. If you don't believe me, I have the paintings to prove it!

July, 2002

INCENTIVES

I've never been much of an antique collector, but there is one antique that quietly rests on a book shelf in my office. It's an ornately framed "Physician's Prayer," that spent the better part of the 1900's on the office wall of a physician who practiced medicine in Vermont for 60 years.

When the elderly general practitioner retired and moved to Pennsylvania, I had the honor of serving as his physician. In the process of rendering medical care to the doctor and his wife, I got to know their family quite well.

On a number of different occasions, I listened to his children reminisce about their father making winter house calls on snow shoes, delivering his own grandchildren, and appreciating a badly-needed Sunday afternoon nap. I also listened to stories about his concerned daughter routinely disconnecting the telephone, thereby facilitating her father's badly-needed naps.

When the doctor died at the age of 95, his family gave me their father's cherished antique. I look at it every time I'm in my office, and when I do, I think about what it must have been like being a physician a half-century ago.

For one thing, physicians had different incentives back then. Their careers were more secure, their place in society was more clearly defined, and their patients were generally more grateful, more understanding, and more supportive.

Physicians were motivated to make middle-of-the night house calls, offer a fuller range of medical and surgical services, and even invent cures a half-century ago because society had different expectations of its physicians. A half-century ago, when a physician did the best he could for a patient, he was sincerely thanked and justifiably praised.

Just as physicians had different incentives, so too did their patients. In an age when specialty medicine, sophisticated technology, and wonder drugs were still waiting to be developed, patients placed a greater amount of trust in their physicians.

A half-century ago, patients were able to engage in good-faith relationships with their doctors because they had a greater understanding of the limitations of medicine. They respected their doctors for their education and dedication, but they also got to know their doctors as friends and neighbors who, like all other human beings, could only do so much.

This highly personal doctor-patient relationship helped ensure a physician's professional as well as financial success. Through direct cash payment, delayed though it may sometimes have been, or the bartering of goods and services, physicians were reimbursed for their services and able to maintain comfortable lifestyles.

Significantly, patients were able to obtain medical care which, by most economic standards, was considered affordable. A half-century ago, patients paid for their medical care as they could and when they could and, somehow, the medical practices of most physicians still managed to stay afloat.

As time marched on, someone got the bright idea that patients could make periodic payments into a general fund, and that payment for their future medical and surgical care could be "insured" through such a fund. As the health insurance industry began to develop, government got a similar notion and began to sponsor its own health insurance programs.

In its infancy, the health insurance industry had different incentives that more closely paralleled those of physicians and patients. Patients' medical bills were paid, physicians were fairly reimbursed, and through the development of a reasonable profit structure, the health insurance industry managed to grow.

In its infancy, government-sponsored health insurance programs also had different incentives that more closely paralleled the needs of society. Health care for the poor and elderly was guaranteed through and financed by a considerate government that initially seemed grateful for the understanding and support of America's physicians.

A lot has changed in the past half-century. Medical care in the United States has undergone a dramatic metamorphosis, and in many ways, many of our health care incentives have been replaced by health care disincentives.

For starters, physicians have less incentive to go out of their way for patients and have very little incentive to attempt any professional heroics. Patients have grown very intolerant of therapeutic maloccurrence, and instead of rendering gratitude and praise for a physician's best efforts, they have turned to malpractice suits and license revocation proceedings.

Additionally, unreasonable reimbursement from managed care, spending cuts in government-sponsored health care programs, government prohibitions against physicians acting as Good Samaritans, an ever-increasing cost of operating a medical practice, and continuing legislative and judicial discrimination against the American medical profession have given physicians less reason to do more. Well-meaning professionals who are frequently treated like criminals and who risk the loss of their personal fortune with every therapeutic intervention have very little incentive to perform optimally.

Similarly, today's patients have less incentive to be more understanding of and cooperative with the entire health care experiment. In many ways, today's patients feel betrayed.

A half-century ago, patients knew their only doctor as a friend and neighbor who could be easily contacted in time of need. Today, patients know all about the training, experience, and publications of each of their various specialists, but they know very little about the families, avocations, or personal needs of these same individuals.

Today, patients feel betrayed by a health care system that replaces physicians with answering services and nurse practitioners. Patients feel betrayed by a system that would substitute a theoretical team of unavailable specialists for an available, affable, and able friend.

Patients feel betrayed by a system that rations health care, makes health care unaffordable, and discourages attempts at preserving America's traditional doctor-patient relationship. It's little wonder that today's health care consumers are angry, frustrated, and quick to blame the closest available representative of the health care industry.

Believe it or not, our current health insurance industry also has less incentive to finance the health care of its beneficiaries. Simply stated, insurance companies charge patients premiums which they invest; health care benefits are paid from interest earned on invested premiums.

By denying health care benefits or by rationing health care, the insurance companies keep a greater amount of money invested which allows a greater amount of compound interest to accrue. This results in greater corporate profits which translates into yearly multi-million dollar performance bonuses for the executives who shape corporate policy and who maintain a healthy corporate bottom line.

Money paid out in health insurance benefits is money that can never become a performance bonus or positively affect an insurance corporation's P/E ratio in the stock market. Herein lies the major disincentive.

Similarly, government also has less incentive to finance health care for the poor and elderly. Entitlement programs have fallen into disfavor with many taxpayers, and taxpayer unrest portends voter unrest, which frequently translates into a swift and permanent transfer of political power.

In this election year, tax cuts and balanced budgets have become key issues for elected officials who want to stay elected. As a result, government's funding of health care for the poor and elderly is being critically evaluated by a large clump of worried politicians.

Our government is run by elected officials who ultimately must answer to the voters. With a substantial number of influential voters and special interest groups demanding tax breaks and an immediate reduction of the federal deficit, government disincentives to providing health care to the poor and elderly abound.

A half-century ago, a humble country doctor walked the less-traveled roads of Vermont. Armed with a pair of snow shoes, a black bag, and a "Physician's Prayer," he answered his calling and provided medical care for the sick and dying.

A half-century ago, this dedicated physician managed to successfully combat disease with fewer treatments, fewer tools, and fewer tests than physicians routinely use today. It's amazing what someone can accomplish with the right incentives.

January, 1996

SMOKE GETS IN YOUR EYES

F red always thought of me as his friend first and his doctor second. That's probably why he waited for me to go on vacation before committing suicide.

He probably figured that he would be dead and buried before I got back, and by that time, I would have gotten the rest I needed. Fred knew how hard I worked at trying to keep him and the rest of my patients alive and well, and I have no doubt that he was as concerned about me as I was about him.

Fred, who had smoked three packs of cigarettes a day for most of his seventy years on this earth, was dying of end stage lung disease the last time I saw him in my office. As he fumbled with the nasal cannula from his portable oxygen unit, he tried to intersperse short phrases between shorter labored breaths.

His ribs retracted forty times a minute as he tried to convince me that he wouldn't be dying if he had met me six years sooner and followed my advice to quit smoking. As he struggled to speak, he stared at me through the eyes of a man who seemed to realize that there were more filter tips in a single carton of cigarettes than there were days remaining in his fragile life.

As busy physicians, we sometimes lose sight of the fact that medicine is more than just matching the treatment from Column A with the disease from Column B, or being able to impress medical residents with the fact that rib retractions and pulsus paradoxus are positively correlated. Sometimes, we lose sight of the responsibility that each of us has to our patients, profession, and society.

For reasons that have more to do with economics than medicine, cigarette smoking is still tolerated in the United States today. Also tolerated are the cancer, emphysema, coronary vascular disease, and incredible host of other maladies that are both actively and passively caused by cigarette smoke.

The time has come for all of us who practice medicine to stop being so tolerant and to start fighting for legal, legislative, and societal changes that will dramatically curtail, if not eliminate, the use of tobacco products in the United States by the end of this century. The time has come for physicians to start practicing preventive medicine where tobacco use is concerned.

It doesn't take too vivid an imagination to realize that the United States could eliminate the vast majority of its tobacco crops and subsidize tobacco farmers to grow other crops that could be used to help feed the many Americans who go to bed hungry every night. These crops could also be sold for profit to help eliminate hunger in other countries.

Tobacco products could then be taxed to make their purchase prohibitive in the United States, and laws could be enacted to make tobacco use illegal in all but private residences. Special provisions could be incorporated into these laws to protect children and the elderly from exposure to tobacco smoke even in private homes.

I feel like George Orwell suggesting the forced elimination of what many consider to be an inherent American birth right, but if we realistically think that we can put an end to drug abuse or drunk driving, we first have to prove that we can put an end to a seemingly tamer national habit that has been taking many more lives for many more years. The elimination of tobacco use in the United States is realistic and necessary, especially since it would dramatically reduce a wide variety of disease processes and help eliminate health care spending for both self-induced and acquired illnesses.

In addition, the substitution of alternate crops for tobacco would help put an end to world hunger, and at the same time, contribute to the American economy. The savings in health care costs and the profits from the sale of alternate crops would help offset financial losses sustained by the tobacco industry.

I know all about the propensity of American law to sacrifice the interests of many to protect the so-called rights of a few, but I also know that smokers don't have the natural right to pollute the air that non-smokers have to breathe. I'm not even sure that smokers have the moral right to harm themselves in more ways than they seem to realize or care to admit.

It's curious how we institutionalize patients with the potential for suicide and incarcerate murderers, and yet continue to tolerate those who are slowly killing themselves and others with cigarette smoke. It's also curious how we continue to tolerate the deleterious effects of tobacco smoke when a wealth of proven scientific fact would support its immediate elimination.

I find some comfort in the fact that I did everything humanly possible to ease Fred's suffering while he was alive, but I'm still troubled by the fact that the ravaging effects of cigarette smoke may one day make the life of another patient or friend intolerable. I never saw Fred's suicide coming, but neither do the many people who tolerate the smoking of a friend or loved one without realizing that they are witnessing a suicide in progress.

The time has come for every American physician to stop ignoring the obvious and do everything in our collective power to remove the deathly stench of tobacco smoke from the air we breathe. If he were still alive, Fred would agree.

January, 1991

A DAY IN THE LIFE

There comes a day each spring that signals the official start of rural Northeastern Pennsylvania's five-month mowing season. For nearly two decades, I have greeted the day with mixed emotions.

To be sure, I enjoy hopping on my lawn tractor every few weeks and mowing the grass on the non-wooded portion of the fourteen acres I call home. Feeling the warm sun and gentle breeze on my face, hearing the rippling brook and animals frolicking in the woods, and smelling the fresh honeysuckle and blooming lilac never fails to awaken those senses that seem to grow dormant each winter.

What churns my emotions is the prospect of hopping on a lawn tractor that invariably finds some way of breaking down the first time it is used each year. Much like a dancing bear that has forgotten how to polka following a long hibernation, every lawn tractor I have ever owned seems to have forgotten how to work properly following a winter in storage.

A number of neighbors have commented that my choice of lawn tractors seems to be the reason for my dilemma. They have observed that a man of my stature should be riding a $5,000 John Deere lawn tractor as opposed to the $1,000 generic model I have become accustomed to buying.

These individuals have argued that a more reputable lawn tractor would provide a decade of predictable service and still have trade-in value. To my way of thinking, however, five years of semi-predictable service at one-fifth the price translates into more bang for the buck.

The principles of lawn tractor economy notwithstanding, the first day of this year's mowing season started off in a relatively painless manner. Following a battery recharge, the repair of a flat tire, and an oil change and lube job, I was riding my lawn tractor and successfully convincing myself that the preliminary effort was a small price to pay for a peaceful and relaxing Saturday afternoon.

After a few laps around my front lawn, my wife signaled that I had an important phone call. Sensing a certain urgency in her signal, I shut off the tractor and made my way to the nearest phone.

The call was from an old friend who lived in another town an hour or so away. With obvious concern, he informed me that his wife had fallen a few weeks earlier sustaining a herniated lumbar disc, was in excruciating pain, and was not tolerating or being helped by her pain medications.

To complicate matters, her personal physician was on vacation, and the specialist she had been referred to for a nerve block could not see her for another month. Adding insult to injury, she was informed that the specialist did not accept her health insurance and that she would have to pay cash at the time of her visit.

When he asked for my advice, I instructed my friend to bring his wife to my home/office as soon as possible. When he noted that I was not on his HMO's list of participating physicians, I told him that I would gladly exchange a medical exam and nerve block for a compliment, sincere or other, on the impending beauty of my lawn, and a reminder of what a great basketball player I was in high school.

Returning to my lawn tractor, I quickly became aware of the fact that its battery was dead. As I proceeded to recharge the battery for the second time in as many hours, I was once again summoned to the phone.

This call was from the wife of a 50 year-old patient who was experiencing chest pain at work. She informed me that her husband, who is hypertensive, diabetic, and hyperlipidemic, was experiencing pain; possibly from strained chest wall muscles; dyspnea and diaphoresis, possibly from the heat of the day; and nausea, possibly from skipping lunch.

When she told me that his pulse was regular and his blood pressure slightly elevated and that his supervisors had advised him to rest for a while, I instructed her to immediately call an ambulance and have her husband transported to the nearest hospital for cardiac evaluation. When she told me that the fellow worker who had taken her husband's vital signs said that he appeared to be stable and possibly even improving, I repeated my instructions and stressed the urgency of the transfer.

Returning again to my tractor, I realized that its old battery was not accepting a new charge. Also realizing that the mowing season was just beginning, I decided to drive into town to buy the battery I should have purchased a few hours earlier.

Following an exchange of batteries, I returned to the task at hand. After only a few more laps around my front lawn, I saw a 1987 Ford sedan pull into my driveway, and my friend and his ailing wife hobble out of the car.

A greeting, a quick shower, and a few phone calls later, I examined my friend's wife, performed a nerve block, and wrote out prescriptions for a few medications and orders for physical therapy. As my wife invited our friends in for lunch, I excused myself and returned to my tractor.

Making up for lost time, I raced around the front lawn and mowed grass with wild abandon. Following lunch with my friends, I returned to the lawn that would be a race track, only to have my mission quickly thwarted by the smell of burning rubber and the sound of a snapping tractor belt.

As I removed the mowing deck from the tractor, I quickly discovered that a new belt had been destroyed because a plastic idler pulley had fractured and malfunctioned. With little recourse, I started calling every hardware, auto parts, and lawn and garden store within a one-hour radius in search of a 3.5 O.D. flat idler pulley.

Somewhere amidst my futile phone search, I received a phone call from my oldest son who was halfway through a 2-day scuba diving certification exam in Virginia. He called because his diving partner started experiencing severe pain and drainage of brown fluid from one of his ears following their first dive.

Although his partner insisted that the fluid was probably just cerumen, that the pain was starting to subside, and that he didn't want to miss the next day's dive, I advised my son to drive his friend to the nearest emergency room for evaluation of what I believed to be hemorrhaging through a ruptured tympanic membrane. Requiring no further discussion, my son followed my advice.

Following my final unsuccessful attempts to locate an idler pulley, I came to the realization that my lawn would have to wait until the necessary part could be ordered and my tractor repaired. I also came to the realization that I had very little to show for the day's lawn mowing efforts.

Later that evening, as I relaxed and reflected on the events of the day, I thought about the people I had helped in between my various attempts at mowing a lawn and repairing a tractor. Although I was not one penny richer for my day's efforts as a physician, I felt amply rewarded by the trust people place in me and by my ability to respond to that trust without regard to financial consequence.

A few days have passed since the start of mowing season. My lawn still looks like a boot camp haircut, and my garage floor is still cluttered with various parts that once combined to create a functioning lawn tractor.

On a brighter note, I just received a phone call from my son who informed me that his diving partner was grateful for my advice, and that his ruptured tympanic membrane is starting to heal nicely. Earlier today, I received a bouquet of flowers from my friend's wife with the message that she was walking better and that her back pain had decreased dramatically.

My patient's wife also called today to inform me that her husband underwent successful coronary artery bypass grafting this morning and to thank me for insisting on a quick ambulance ride to the hospital. It seems that work, the weather, and missing lunch had very little to do with his recent symptoms, and that timely medical care helped save his life.

Reflecting on a day in the life of a doctor reveals many a truth and raises one of the most important questions of our time. Does anyone know where I can find a 3.5 O.D. flat idler pulley?

May, 2000

ADVENTURES IN PSYCHOTHERAPY

W.R. Kasey is a clinical psychologist—and a good one at that! He is also a caring and compassionate human being.

His only real shortcoming is in the area of music appreciation. W.R. truly believes that *Time Of The Season* by the Zombies had a greater impact on the history of music than *Good Vibrations* by the Beach Boys!

Like many of us, W.R. came up the hard way. He worked his way through college and graduate school, and after receiving his doctorate, he completed an internship in clinical psychology at a university hospital.

For the past few years, he has been running an intern training program in clinical psychology. To augment his modest income, he has also been serving as a consultant at an inner city psychiatric center.

W.R. works hard at what he does. He has grown accustomed to long hours and unexpected emergencies.

He frequently talks about getting away to the mountains for a weekend with his family, but more often than not, his work keeps him close to home. Like many other dedicated clinical psychologists, W.R. is a valuable resource to the medical profession.

Recently, a 45 year-old patient told me about her experiences with a different breed of psychologist. Our discussion made me realize the dangers of professional inbreeding.

Unlike W.R., this self-proclaimed "psychotherapist" does not have his doctorate in psychology. Instead, he has a master's degree in social work, but since he passed the appropriate examination, he has been licensed to provide psychotherapeutic services to patients in New York State.

Unlike W.R., he does not work in a facility where back-up from psychiatrists or psychologists are mandated or readily available. Instead, he works alone—in the seclusion of his own office.

For approximately 2 months, Connie, who was experiencing a mid-life crisis and marital problems, consulted this therapist. Initially, she was given one-hour appointments twice weekly, but after a few weeks, one of the private appointments was replaced by a weekly group therapy session.

During her first visit, Connie was informed that her husband would also require psychotherapy. However, Connie's husband refused.

Each of Connie's private sessions cost $85, and each group therapy session cost $45. She was required to pay cash at the time of each session, but was told that the therapist "was recognized" by every insurance company.

As Connie later discovered, the therapist may have been recognized by every insurance company, but not as anyone whose professional services were likely to be covered by health insurance. Connie was understandably angry over the fact that she had to pay $800 out of her own pocket for sessions the therapist initially said would be covered by her health insurance.

She was also angry over the fact that the therapist had been recommended to her by a medical professional—her gynecologist. She was angry over just about everything else she saw.

During her private sessions with the therapist, Connie felt like she was talking to the wall. The therapist doodled and continually checked his watch while Connie poured out her heart.

On multiple occasions, the therapist told his very attractive patient that her progress in therapy might be accelerated by one of his special group trips to the Caribbean. He told her that he took a group of special patients to the Caribbean every 3 months and that he generally found group therapy and private counseling to be more effective when offered in a relaxed tropical atmosphere!

Connie was also angry over what she saw in group therapy. She saw a large number of pathetic patients who were willing to pay $45 just to have someone to talk to on a weekly basis.

She saw patients who had been referred because of intractable pain, patients who had been referred because of uncontrollable neurotic behavior, and patients who had been referred because of psychotic tendencies. She saw patients who had been in the same group for 5 years, patients who did not know if psychotherapy was helping them, and patients who came back every week because they didn't know what else to do.

Connie did not understand why so many different patients with so many different problems were all receiving the same therapy. She admitted that everyone felt good when they physically took their anger out on a large, stuffed dummy, but she did not understand why everyone was required to stand up and shout personalized expletives at every other member of the group.

There was a lot about her brief excursion into psychotherapy that Connie did not understand. That is why she left the process after only 2 months.

To say that Connie did not get anything out of her therapy sessions would be misleading because she was able to put her own problems into perspective by witnessing the profound suffering of some of the other people in her group. She was also able to get past being "in therapy," a hurdle which too many people in Connie's generation seem obliged to overcome on their way to self-actualization.

In the United States today, there are many skilled individuals who are able to provide valuable therapy and counseling services. Most of these individuals are employed by agencies that also employ psychiatrists and psychologists to provide optimal care for the patients they serve.

There are also an alarming number of inadequately-trained individuals who are allowed to work without supervision and who use their professional licenses as tickets for a ride on the gravy train of human emotion. No one group or profession can claim exclusivity where problems of the human psyche are concerned, but some problems are better served by trained psychologists rather than travel agents who are masquerading as such.

It is important for physicians and their patients to become familiar with the various psychiatric and psychological services in their communities. A rose may be a rose, but a psychotherapist may not be a psychotherapist.

It is also important for all of us in the medical profession to voice our opposition to the growing tendency of many state licensing boards to transfer important functions from Medicine's exclusive domain to that of other professions. Counselors should not be allowed to diagnose and treat patients with severe psychiatric problems in an unsupervised environment any more than pharmacists should be allowed to prescribe drugs for their customers.

Connie has come a long way since her husband took her on a second honeymoon to the Caribbean, and our medical staff is currently investigating the therapeutic effects of shouting expletives at each other during medical staff meetings! Now, if we can only figure out a way to get W.R. to stop singing **She Drives Me Crazy** while making rounds on the Psychiatry ward!

June, 1991

THE QUALITY OF MERCY

While traveling through the Australian outback, a group of weary hikers stumbled upon a trading post near the small town of Mersey. When the hikers entered the establishment and requested a round of cold drinks, they were served tall glasses of iced tea.

As they began to savor the refreshing tea, one of the hikers made a number of unusual facial contortions and attempted to remove debris from his tongue.

"Is something wrong with your drink, Mate?" the store owner inquired.

"No," the hiker replied. "The tea's alright, but there's hair in my glass."

"Why, that's the secret ingredient what gives the tea its unusual taste," the store owner commented.

"What ingredient might that be?" the hiker asked, as he continued to remove small hairs from his tongue.

"Well, if you must know," the store owner replied, "the secret ingredient is fur from a koala bear. Everyone in these parts sprinkles a bit of koala fur in their tea to give it flavor."

As the remaining hikers inspected their drinks, one of them asked the store owner if he ever considered pouring the tea through a strainer before serving.

"Oh, no, Mate, I couldn't do that," the store owner replied. "The koala tea of Mersey is not strained!

In his classic, **The Merchant Of Venice**, William Shakespeare taught us that the quality of mercy is not strained. Through the character of Portia, the Bard showed us that mercy is natural, spontaneous, and intact, rather than forced, processed, or diluted.

In recent months, a number of articles and letters concerning pro bono medical care in the managed care setting have been published in various medical journals. Most of these articles have contended that managed care has made pro bono medical care difficult, if not impossible, to render.

Instead of dealing with the quality of mercy, these articles have dealt with the quantity of remuneration. In doing so, they have aptly demonstrated health care's ominous metamorphosis from a quality-based medical model to a quantity-based business model.

It is true that managed care has led to a reduction in income for many physicians, as well increased time constraints for many others. This might explain why certain physicians feel that they no longer have the time or financial wherewithal to provide pro bono medical care to the poor and needy.

Unfortunately, managed care has also led to the removal of freedom from far too many medical practices. This might explain why so many physicians have been forced to march lockstep to the beat of managed care rather than to a more personal beat that originates in one's own heart.

Providing medical care to the poor and needy has always been one of the medical profession's most important responsibilities. Managed care's shameless abrogation of that responsibility has sent a loud and clear message that there is no place for charity or mercy in the new business of medicine.

One need only review the track record of the Medicare HMOs to see how managed care routinely abandons the financially disadvantaged. Managed care organizations have cancelled the health insurance of Medicare patients by the tens-of-thousands in unprofitable geographic locations and then moved on to other markets where equal numbers of elderly patients were unwittingly subjected to similar fates.

Managed care has always and will always be about quantity. It is quantity that motivates managed care's executives, guarantees profits for its organizations, and keeps its stockholders happy.

Medicine, on the other hand, has always been about quality. It is medicine's quality, including its quality of mercy that has helped define the profession.

Adhering to a strict business model, managed care has ensured quantity by forcing medicine to sacrifice quality. Aye, there's the rub!

Early in my medical career, I discovered the futility of having to bill Medicaid three separate times for a payment of $6. I found it much easier to provide medical care without charge to an occasional patient than to play the exasperating games of health insurers who were better at denying medical services than they were at paying for them.

When I finally received $6 from Medicaid six months after rendering medical care to a patient, the payment was meaningless. When I rendered medical care to a patient without expectation of payment, the benefits to my self-esteem, my patients, and my profession were immediate and substantial.

Throughout my medical career, I have provided pro bono medical care to patients who were out of work, to the poor and uninsured, and to needy patients whose insurance payments didn't cover the cost of filing an insurance claim. In all honesty, providing such care has never interfered with my ability to earn a comfortable living as a physician or, for that matter, to turn out the lights in my office after I was finished with my final patient of the day.

The poor and the needy should not be abandoned just to safeguard managed care's profit structure. Perhaps managed care should be abandoned to safeguard the right of physicians to participate in one of their profession's most noble, most necessary, and most rewarding activities.

The quality of mercy is not strained. For that matter, neither is the koala tea of Mersey!

June, 1999

ABORTIONS

By the time she entered her teens, Meg had already been raped by her guardian-uncle on multiple separate occasions. When she became pregnant, her uncle, who was the corrupt mayor of a small town, sent her away for an abortion.

Returning home, she experienced vaginal bleeding, and was taken to see the town's general practitioner. The doctor, who was never apprised of the attempted abortion, was able to stop the hemorrhaging, and report to her family that Meg was pregnant.

When he learned that the attempted abortion had failed, her uncle arranged for Meg to receive pre-natal care, and for her baby to be given up for adoption at birth. He also arranged for a teenage boy to take the rap for Meg's pregnancy, and for the boy's entire family to be run out of town.

For many years, Meg lived with the fear of being killed if she ever revealed her uncle's shameless indiscretions. She also lived with the sorrow of a young mother who had never seen her baby.

Fortunately, she was able to deal with her early-life misfortunes in a constructive manner and complete her education. It time, Meg was able to successfully handle a number of different business ventures and become a highly respected member of the business community.

Many years later, Meg married and became pregnant, but during the pregnancy, her diabetes became very difficult to control, her osteoarthritis became unbearably painful, and she became hypertensive. Her obstetrician advised abortion, but Meg decided to see the pregnancy through, and ultimately gave birth to a healthy daughter.

Since the Supreme Court decided ***Roe vs. Wade*** and legalized abortion in the United States, Pro-Choice advocates have argued that pregnancy resulting from incest or rape, as well as pregnancy that threatened the health and/or life of the mother, were clear-cut indications for abortion. Unfortunately, the Pro-Choice camp has conveniently disregarded the fact that pregnancy following incest or rape is so statistically insignificant that it borders on the non-existent, that high-risk pregnancy centers have made the treatment of complicated pregnancies routine, and that abortion is nothing less than the willful destruction of unborn human life.

An ensemble of Hollywood starlets can talk all about their right to determine what happens inside their bodies, but the unborn also have rights. The use of abortion as a means of birth control or as a way to select future progeny on the basis of sex or astrological sign are flagrant violations of these rights.

In many ways, abortion is the inevitable consequence of a society that has worked hard at developing a "throw-away" mentality. We think nothing of throwing away our empty soda bottles and our old cars, and, unfortunately, we also think nothing of throwing away our marriages, our families, and the unborn that do not seem to fit into our immediate plans.

It was not too many years ago that America underwent an unprecedented sexual revolution. Unfortunately, too many Americans celebrated their new sexual freedom without realizing that new freedom mandates new responsibility.

AIDS and other sexually-transmitted diseases are examples of what this oversight has already cost our nation. Abortion is another.

No one can condone incest or rape, just as no one can condone the return of the back alley butcher shops where amateur abortionists routinely injured young women who were attempting to terminate their unwanted pregnancies. What all of us can condone, however, is a new respect for life and a fuller understanding of the miracle that too many people take for granted and too many people thoughtlessly destroy.

As the Supreme Court once again considers the issue of abortion, our nation needs a wake-up call and a reminder that is it senseless to help create human life only to later aid in its destruction. As a society, we need to become Pre-Choice, rather than Pro-Choice, and give serious consideration to all the ramifications of pregnancy before it occurs.

A few years ago, Meg received a phone call from a young man who identified himself as a social worker who specialized in adoption services for pregnant women and social services for single mothers. He told Meg that he was in the middle of a research project and that he wanted to meet with her and discuss her teenage pregnancy.

Throughout their phone conversation, the social worker stressed how his research would be greatly facilitated by a better understanding of how Meg's child was taken away from her at birth. At first, Meg was reluctant to meet with the young man, but when he explained how much work had already been done to locate someone with her unique history, she finally agreed.

When the young social worker came to Meg's door for their first meeting, he smiled, handed her his business card, and said, "Hi, Mom, remember me?" Countless hugs and tears later, the young social worker told his mother the long story of the lifetime search that finally allowed them to be reunited for the first time since his birth.

Life is truly a matter of perspective. And without life, perspective is inconsequential.

June, 1992

THE PAST AS PROLOGUE

An old legend resurfaced recently in *Chicken Soup For The Soul.* Tis' a moral tale that bears repeating.

In the late 1800's, a British lord took his family to Scotland for a vacation. The holiday nearly ended in tragedy when his adventurous young son wandered off into the woods alone and decided to test the waters of a secluded swimming hole.

When the young boy experienced severe abdominal cramps and struggled to stay afloat in the water, he cried out for help. Fortunately, a farm boy working in a nearby field heard the cries and was able to respond in time to save the drowning lad.

When he learned about the incident, the British lord traveled to the farm boy's home to personally thank the young hero for saving his son's life. During the course of their meeting, the lord discovered that the farm boy dreamed of becoming a doctor, but was unable to pursue the necessary course of study because of his family's poverty.

In gratitude for the farm boy's heroics, the lord offered to pay for his medical education. Wisely, the youngster took advantage of the generous offer, and in time, was awarded a medical degree from St. Mary's Hospital in London.

Decades later, Winston Churchill developed life-threatening pneumonia while traveling through North Africa. Dr. Alexander Fleming, who had just recently discovered a wonder drug called penicillin, was summoned.

Responding immediately, Dr. Fleming administered penicillin to Prime Minister Churchill, and saved his life—for the second time. Many years earlier, it was the farm boy, Alexander Fleming, who responded to the cries of a drowning child and saved the life of young Winston Churchill!

Today, far too many stories are being written about physicians who have become disenchanted with the medical profession or our current health care delivery system and have decided to take an early retirement or pursue other professional interests outside the field of medicine. Not enough stories are being written about the countless individuals who continue to dream, as Alexander Fleming once did, of becoming a doctor.

Today, far too many articles are being published about physicians attempting to defraud Medicare, Medicaid, and everyone else who pays health care bills. Not enough articles are being published about the hundreds of thousands of American physicians who help educate young doctors by generously contributing to colleges, universities, and medical schools, just as Lord Randolph Churchill once did; who help train future physicians by serving as unpaid teachers and preceptors; and who provide pro bono health care to the poor.

Today, too many stories are being told about physicians who are incompetent, impaired, or unable to tell the difference between acceptable medical care and malpractice. Not enough stories are being told about the daily heroics of hundreds of thousands of American physicians—heroics that, in many instances, would easily rival those of Alexander Fleming.

Today, too many slings and arrows are being shot at the American medical profession for problems that were created, not by physicians, but by crooked politicians, greedy businessmen, and low-flying legal eagles. Too few wreaths are being handed to the multitude of physicians whose ongoing fight against human suffering continues to shape the course of history in ways no less significant than Fleming's emergency care of Churchill in the early 1940's.

Today, children and young adults still dream of becoming doctors. In more cases than not, they dream, not of discovering miracle cures or taking care of celebrities, but of following in the footsteps of physicians whose names and practice locations are generally unfamiliar to all but the patients whose lives they've touched.

Today, these dreamers still turn into doctors who become benefactors, unsung heroes, and shapers of history. What's more, they also become active participants in the process of healing.

In recent years, physicians have become the target of bad press and innuendo, and the victims of socialized medicine, but the fundamentals of the medical profession have remained essentially unchanged. People still get sick and turn to their doctors for help, and regardless of what politicians, lawyers, or health insurers have to say about the matter, doctors continue to provide the help their patients require.

The past is prologue, and society's reawakening to the importance of its healers is imminent. In the meantime, an inspirational tale will help take the chill out of the soul—and a cup of chicken soup couldn't hurt either!

April, 1999

ALZHEIMER'S DISEASE

I t was not the kind of day two people would care to remember as their 50th wedding anniversary. Ted was experiencing the combined effects of fatigue and pain from his chronic anemia and osteoarthritis, and Jenny was experiencing the chronic fear and bewilderment of a person who was being held captive inside her own body.

When Jenny sustained multiple injuries after unexpectedly wandering away from a family celebration and falling, a "Golden Anniversary" suddenly lost some of its luster. The occurrence made everyone realize that certain diseases affect families and communities as much as they do individual patients.

Jenny is one of over 4-million Americans afflicted with Alzheimer's disease. As such, she is a member of a group that currently includes 10% of all Americans over the age of 65, and 50% of all Americans over the age of 85.

Although hard to imagine, the number of Americans with Alzheimer's disease is expected to quadruple within the next 50 years. When viewed in light of America's increasing life expectancy, such a projection becomes especially ominous.

To date, the cause of Alzheimer's disease is still a mystery. Although genetic susceptibility is suggested by the discovery of a familial form of Alzheimer's and by the predictable occurrence of Alzheimer's disease in the vast majority of patients with Down's syndrome who survive past the age of 40, non-genetic causes have also been postulated.

Environmental toxins, such as aluminum, have also been suggested as possible etiological agents. Furthermore, studies demonstrating that neurological abnormalities can be induced in a high percentage of laboratory animals by injecting them with white blood cells taken from close contacts of patients with Alzheimer's disease have led researchers to postulate that the disease may be caused by the human-to-human transmission of a slow virus, as in the case of other dementing illnesses, such as kuru and Creutzfeldt-Jakob disease.

In the United States today, Alzheimer's disease has become the 4th leading cause of death among adults, claiming over 100,000 lives yearly. Patients typically live between 5 and 20 years after the disease becomes apparent, with most patients surviving 10 years.

For the families of elderly patients with many chronic diseases, such survival rates would be looked upon with optimism, but Alzheimer's disease has historically provided very little cause for optimism. In the process of slowly losing memory, intellectual capability, and physical well-being, a patient with Alzheimer's disease requires a tremendous amount of care and support.

In many instances, the people who provide care for patients with Alzheimer's disease are also elderly patients with health care problems of their own. Insofar as Medicare does not pay for custodial care, and Medicaid only pays for such care after a patient's financial resources have been totally depleted, the onus of caring for patients with Alzheimer's disease has fallen on spouses and families.

In the United States today, 3 out of 4 Alzheimer's patients are currently being managed at home. Predictably, the stress of such management has caused a dramatic increase in the number of illnesses among those who are charged with their care.

Just as Alzheimer's disease is a source of constant frustration to the families of its victims, it is also frustrating to those of us who attempt to manage a disease we don't understand with treatments we don't have. We are still waiting for FDA approval of THA, or tacrine, which may prove effective in the treatment of the disease but which appears to be limited by its potential for hepatotoxicity.

Other Alzheimer's drugs are also being developed at the present time. Unlike THA, however, most of these drugs are not being "fast-tracked" by the FDA and still appear to be light years away.

It would appear that the first step in conquering Alzheimer's disease will have to come from the federal government. Before we can figure out how to treat or prevent Alzheimer's disease, we must first figure out what it is and from where it comes.

This will require research, and research will require money. Unfortunately, any understanding of Alzheimer's disease and any development of effective treatment will require a great deal of research which, in turn, will require a great deal of funding.

In 1991, the federal government will pay the National Institutes of Health $230-million for Alzheimer's research. As federal spending goes, this is a mere drop in the bucket.

With $230-million, the federal government could only add 2 more F-117A Stealth Fighters to our current collection, bail out our Savings and Loan industry for about 15 minutes, or insult a foreign aid-seeking nation, thereby endangering our "favorite lender" status within the international community. If serious Alzheimer's research is going to be done, the federal government has to start coming up with some serious money.

It would also appear that the federal and state governments are going to have to create programs that help with the home care of Alzheimer's patients. Day care programs and ancillary service programs are desperately needed by those who care for Alzheimer's patients, and with a little imagination, one social service project might be creatively used to help another.

Healthy, unemployed recipients of public assistance could be trained to help with the care of Alzheimer's patients, as well as with elderly patients who have other illnesses, thereby providing the elderly and infirm the help they need and welfare recipients with gainful employment and the ability to contribute to society. Significantly, this could all be done without any additional expenditure by federal or state governments.

Finally, it is obvious that progress against Alzheimer's disease is not going to be made without effective drugs. THA may be such a drug.

THA release is being currently held up by the FDA because of the drug's propensity to cause a dose-related, but reversible, elevation of liver enzymes. At this point in time, the release of THA would appear to be warranted on the basis of the extraordinary need of a drug for use in Alzheimer's disease.

If THA's potential for hepatic injury is the major concern of the FDA, it should be remembered that common drugs, such as: methyldopa, isoniazid, acetaminophen, phenytoin, salicylates, methotrexate, quinidine, tetracycline, chlorpromazine, erythromycin estolate, sulfonamides, gold, anabolic steroids and oral contraceptives, can also cause hepatic injury but are still widely and safely used. It should also be remembered that one of our major hepatotoxins, alcohol, is consumed in great quantity worldwide, and can be readily obtained without a prescription.

Only widespread clinical use will be able to assess THA's value and safety in the treatment of Alzheimer's disease. Obviously, such use cannot start without FDA approval.

I saw Ted and Jenny a few days ago. Ted is still weak and arthritic although he refuses to admit as much, and Jenny continues to view the world, which she seems to be slowly fading away from, with a vacuous stare.

I have done everything I can to ease their suffering, but all I have left to give them is the hope that tomorrow may bring the means by which Alzheimer's disease can be treated and prevented. Sometimes, hope is the only medicine that any of us can prescribe.

August, 1991

RURAL HEALTH CARE

In the 1970's, the complexion of American medical education underwent an unprecedented change. Medical school lecture halls started looking less like National Honor Society convocations and more like auditions for the road company of *Hair,* and medical students started talking less of specialization and more of primary care medicine.

A formidable number of medical students even started talking about moving to the country where it was rumored that physicians practiced medicine by day and sat around camp fires singing John Denver songs and drinking Coor's Beer by night. Yours truly was one of those students.

If I ever had any romantic notions about rural medicine, they were quickly dispelled during my first week of practice in rural Northeastern Pennsylvania, circa 1981. On my first night on call in the emergency room of a small rural hospital, I saw an elderly patient in fulminant congestive heart failure.

When I ordered a stat dose of intravenous furosemide, I was told by the ER nurse that the hospital was temporarily out of the drug. Fortunately, the shock of the nurse's revelation wore off quickly, and I was able to find a few other drugs with which to treat the patient's failing heart.

Later in the same week, I admitted a patient with a pulmonary embolism to the hospital. When I ordered heparin to be administered by a continuous infusion pump, the charge nurse appeared to be confused by the order.

When a complete explanation of an infusion pump's function and a thorough review of all the device's known synonyms failed to alter the

63

nurse's bewildered look, it became apparent that the hospital did not possess any device by which intravenous medications could be continuously administered to a patient. Fortunately, the hospital still had some heparin in its pharmacy, and I was able to anticoagulate the patient by administering the drug every 4 hours.

Today, 10 years later, the same hospital cannot remember the last time it ran out of furosemide or the last time heparin was not administered by a continuous infusion pump. Unfortunately, the same hospital also cannot remember the last time it felt secure about its own existence.

The health care industry has fallen on hard times in the United States, but nowhere more so than in rural America. In the United States today, there are 2.25 physicians for every 1,000 urban residents, but only 1 physician for every 1,000 rural residents.

In fact, well over 100 rural counties in the United States currently have no physician at all. Whereas the urban areas of the country have full complements of primary care physicians and specialists, most rural areas are lucky to have family practitioners and general surgeons, and frequently consider even internists, obstetricians and pediatricians luxury items.

There are many reasons why our rural areas have a difficult time attracting physicians. First of all, the vast majority of American physicians are natives of urban and suburban areas, have very little understanding of this nation's rural areas and residents, and have very little desire to live, work, and raise a family in an isolated and economically-disadvantaged part of the country.

Many physicians truly question what kind of education their children will be able to receive in these areas, what kind of social life and recreation are available, and what kind of professional opportunities await at a small rural hospital with an even smaller medical staff. Physicians generally do not give serious consideration to practicing in the country because rural physicians earn significantly less than their urban counterparts, even though their work schedules frequently rival those of first-year medical residents.

Medicare and other third party payers pay rural physicians less than urban physicians for the same services. Additionally, rural patients are less likely to have health care insurance or to qualify for Medicaid than urban patients, thereby requiring rural physicians to treat a greater percentage of uninsured patients that urban physicians.

The popular belief that country doctors are paid for their medical services with chickens and eggs is generally inaccurate only because many of today's rural patients do not even have the chickens or the eggs with which to barter for medical services. Consequently, many of the services rendered by rural physicians are on a pro bono basis.

Rural areas also have a difficult time attracting physicians because the working conditions of rural physicians are impoverished in comparison to those of urban physicians. Rural hospitals are generally poorly equipped, inadequately staffed, and financially strained.

Rural physicians must rely more on skill and intuition than on sophisticated equipment to make diagnoses, learn how to treat patients with the help of mere skeleton crews of nurses and technicians and without readily-available consultative back-up, and rely on their own ingenuity and resolve when certain drugs and supplies become temporarily unavailable because of a rural hospital's inability to keep up with its bills. In addition, rural physicians are frequently forced to work outside their areas of training and expertise.

Since most rural hospitals cannot afford to employ regular emergency room physicians, they usually require their staff physicians to take emergency room call on a regular basis and frequently pay them only token fees to do so. In this age of specialization, surgeons handling cardiac emergencies and internists handling obstetrical catastrophes are still common occurrences in many rural hospitals.

Unfortunately, such acts of medical heroism often help promote other, more complicated problems. Because of their constant exposure to problems outside their areas of expertise and their relative inability to practice medicine with the same facility and by many of the same standards as their urban counterparts, rural physicians are easy targets for peer reviewers and malpractice lawyers.

Even though many rural hospitals boast exemplary medical staffs with higher percentages of board-certified physicians than many urban medical centers, rural physicians cannot always diagnose and treat patients as quickly and as effectively as physicians who have easy access to state-of-the-art technology and cadres of medical and surgical specialists. Instead of gratitude and recognition for performances above and beyond the call of duty, rural physicians are frequently forced to settle for unfavorable decisions by peer review organizations and courts.

Today, more than ever before, the only thing that rural physicians can be certain of is uncertainty. Over 200 rural hospitals have closed in the past decade, but the mere fact that our remaining rural hospitals are integral parts of this nation's health care delivery system and its rural economy will unlikely be enough to keep their doors open.

Our rural areas are considered political non-entities by many of our legislators because of the sparse number of votes these areas provide, and the health care needs of rural residents are not usually accorded priority status in the federal and state legislatures. If they were, Medicare would not be allowed to pay small rural hospitals $400 less than nearby urban hospitals for the hospitalization of a patient with pneumonia, peer review organizations would not be allowed to prey on rural hospitals so that their action quotas might be met, and an army of unsung rural physicians would not find themselves constantly struggling to earn a living.

With all its inherent problems, practicing medicine in a rural area can still be a highly rewarding experience. I would tell you about all the attractive features of rural medicine but a few of the physicians from a nearby rural hospital are on their way over here for an informal get-together.

One of my guests is bringing a few Spyro Gyra albums and another is picking up a case of early-harvest Riesling from a nearby winery. I hope someone remembers the marshmallows for the camp fire!

September, 1991

WILD BILL AND ROY

Hidden in the office files of one of my patients is a photograph of two men. The first man in the photo would probably not be recognized by most of the people who lived within shouting distance of his home, while the second man would undoubtedly be recognized by millions of people all over the world.

Although the two men traveled widely divergent roads before their brief meeting was preserved in a photo, both had a great deal in common. Both were born and raised in the north before migrating to various points south, both were once employed as fruit pickers, and both were proud to be thought of as cowboys.

Although my patient, Wild Bill, and his friend, Roy, had even more in common, they lived most of their adult lives in two entirely different worlds. Wild Bill's world was one of simplicity and essentials, while Roy's world was one of glamour and riches.

Those who knew Wild Bill understood that his name better reflected who he wanted to be than who he actually was. Wild Bill wanted to be a cowboy, who wore a white hat, rode a magnificent stallion, and packed a pair of glimmering six-shooters.

In reality, though, Wild Bill was a quiet, diminutive man who spent the fifty years of his life co-existing with cerebral palsy, a speech impediment, various crippling injuries, nagging medical conditions, and life-threatening cardiac abnormalities. Boots and saddles occupied little space in Wild Bill's real life, but a prominent space in his dreams.

It's not surprising, then, that Wild Bill idolized "The King of the Cowboys," Roy Rogers, and dreamed of one day meeting his hero. Roy was everything Wild Bill wanted to be—a larger-than-life cowboy who used his healthy body and strong voice to enforce the "Code of the West."

Of course, Roy Rogers won the hearts of senoritas and foiled the bad guys more on the silver screen than in real life, but it was in real life where Roy's star shined the brightest. His movies and television shows were the magnets Roy Rogers used to attract his ardent fans, but it was in his real life meetings with many of these fans—the crippled children, the terminally-ill adults, and the ageless handicapped, where "The Singing Cowboy" made his greatest impact.

Roy Rogers was a straight-shooter and a plain-talker who didn't leave his act in reels of celluloid. In many ways, he was a doctor who used sincere compassion, a friendly voice, and a warm smile to treat the pain and suffering of his unfortunate fans.

Roy Rogers didn't possess a medical degree or a well-stocked pharmacy, and he didn't dispense cures. To his ill and injured patients, he provided something too potent to be bottled and too unique to be synthesized in a laboratory; to those who came seeking his help, Roy Rogers provided the gift of hope.

One of Medicine's most poorly understood phenomena deals with a person's sense of imminent death. By all diagnostic parameters, a patient may be judged to be in good health, but that patient may still sense, and occasionally report, that he or she is dying.

Shortly after his fiftieth birthday, Wild Bill began to sense that he was dying. Despite contrary opinions and reassurances from a number of different cardiologists, Wild Bill felt that he was not long for this world.

Reiterating an earlier vow to meet Roy Rogers before he died, Wild Bill traveled to the California town where his hero lived. Making his presence and intentions known to the owner of a popular restaurant in that town, Wild Bill was told that Roy would be notified pronto that some varmint was looking for him.

The following day, as Wild Bill sipped coffee in the restaurant, he was tapped on the shoulder by an elderly man dressed in conservative

western attire. Although the cowboy's appearance was older than antic-
ipated, his friendly voice and unmistakable smile made Wild Bill
quickly realize that a life-long dream had finally come true, and that he
was actually shaking hands with Roy Rogers.

Following a memorable conversation and a brief photo session,
Wild Bill returned to his winter residence in Florida. A few weeks later,
he died unexpectedly.

After Wild Bill's funeral, his family gave me the photograph he had
taken with Roy Rogers. During many office visits, Wild Bill and I rem-
inisced about Roy Rogers, Dale Evans, Gabby Hayes, The Sons of the
Pioneers, and a horse named, Trigger, and his family knew that the
photograph would hold special meaning for me.

For the past few years, the photograph has been kept in Wild Bill's
office folder. In all honesty, I've looked at the photo on numerous
occasions, and seeing it has never failed to bring a smile to my face or a
number of pertinent concepts to mind.

Whenever I look at the photo of Wild Bill and Roy, I see a little boy
who never grew up, receiving the gift of hope from another little boy
who never grew up. Whenever I look at the photo, I am reminded that
caring is about people and not about pills, diagnostic tests, or health
care delivery systems, and I am humbled by the overwhelming power
of the human spirit.

On July 6, 1998, Roy Rogers died of congestive heart failure at his
home in California. He was 86 years old.

Since his death, he has been remembered, both publicly and pri-
vately, in many different ways. Roy Rogers has been remembered as a
star of the silver screen, a cowboy, a singer, a shrewd businessman, and
a man of fame and fortune.

If a photo in my possession counts for anything, I'd say that Roy
Roger's should also be remembered as an honorary doctor. He treated
fear with a smile, uncertainty with a kind word, and despair with hope.

Many physicians work wonders with their many different medical and surgical skills. Roy Rogers did the same with a therapeutic regimen that always seemed to suggest happy trails.

July, 1998

THE FRUIT AND THE TREE

Somewhere in your many travels, you've probably heard it said that "the fruit doesn't fall far from the tree." This phrase attests to the indisputable fact that children frequently behave like or resemble one or both of their parents.

The parent is the tree and the child is the fruit. The analogy is clear.

A few months ago, I spent a week-end on a college campus with my oldest son, Chris. Having been previously accepted into the college's honors program, he was invited to participate in an essay contest and compete for a four-year, full-tuition scholarship.

If anyone ever wanted to test the premise of fruit not falling far from the tree, all they had to do was observe the way Chris and I handled our week-end together on campus. In appearance, mannerisms, and preferences, Chris and I are as identical as a father and son can be, and our week-end together left at least one college campus with a clearer understanding of applied genetics.

While Chris was writing his essays, I had the opportunity to participate in a number of parent workshops and meet a number of pre-med students. The college students had no idea that I was a physician, and I used my anonymity to help wrest some insights from the doctors of tomorrow.

During one workshop, I asked an unsuspecting pre-med student why he wanted to become a physician.

"Because I want to help people," he answered confidently.

"So, why Medicine?" I inquired. "Couldn't you help people as a social worker, or teacher, or researcher?"

"Sure," he quickly responded, "but I think that I could help them more as a doctor."

"But what about all those long, hard years of training?" I asked. "Is becoming a doctor really worth all the book work, and nights on call, and personal sacrifices?"

"The training's tough, alright," he answered, as though he really understood the untold truths of medical training, "but becoming a doctor is my dream, and I'm not afraid to work hard to make my dream come true."

"What happens if your dream takes you into socialized medicine?" I asked.

"I don't think socialized medicine will ever come to the United States," he responded, "but even if it did, I'd still want to be a doctor and be able to help people."

In the next session, I used a different approach on another unsuspecting pre-med student.

"So, what do you plan to do with all the money you're going to make as a physician?" I asked.

"Oh, I don't know if I'll really make that much money," she replied, with a sheepish smile.

"Well, aren't all doctors millionaires?" I asked. "And don't they all drive Cadillacs and live in mansions?"

"No, that's not true," she replied with a persistent smile. "I live in a rural area and my doctor drives a Bronco and lives on a small farm. I'm pretty sure that he's not a millionaire."

"Now, wait a minute," I continued. "Why would someone spend all those years in college and medical school and residency training if they weren't going to make a lot of money when they finally completed their education?"

"I can't speak for anybody else," she replied calmly, "but money was never the reason I wanted to become a doctor. I want to go back home when my training's finished and practice pediatrics. I want to make enough money so that I can live comfortably, but I'm not worried about getting rich."

"Do you think that managed care will interfere with your ability to earn a decent living or lead to socialized medicine in America?" I asked.

"I don't think so," she replied. "I don't think that the rest of the doctors will let that happen."

In the final workshop, I encountered still another unsuspecting doctor of the future.

"If all these doctors train so hard for so many years, how come so many of them are being sued for malpractice?" I asked.

"I guess society's becoming sue-crazy," she replied with some uncertainty.

"Well, are there so many bad doctors in America?" I inquired.

"I guess there are some bad doctors," she acknowledged, "but I think a lot of good doctors get sued too."

"Why's that?" I asked.

"Probably because some doctors are just the victim of circumstance," she answered, "and probably because there are a lot of lawyers, and it's real easy to sue a doctor."

"Doesn't all this frighten you and make you wonder if all your hard work is really worth the effort?" I asked.

"Not really," she replied. "All I can do is study hard and become the best doctor I can. Then, hopefully, I won't have to worry about malpractice suits and stuff like that."

Following each discussion, I identified myself as a physician, and explained the reasons for my questions. The students seemed relieved to hear that I was a doctor in search of fresh insights, rather than a misinformed parent, and grateful for the opportunity to ask me a few of their own questions about med school, residency programs, and the practice of medicine.

If it's true that the fruit doesn't fall far from the tree, this medical profession of ours still hasn't lost its ability to project a positive image. The pre-med students I recently met, as well as many others I've encountered in my travels, appear to be just as idealistic as we were when we were first preparing to embark on our medical careers, just as industrious, and just as enthusiastic.

Despite talk of an on-going malpractice epidemic, managed care, and the many other woes that are currently befalling the medical profession, these students remain steadfast in their desire to carry on Medicine's time-honored tradition. They've seen America's doctors at work, and they've apparently liked what they've seen.

All of us who practice medicine and teach the art are the branches of a strong tree that has roots extending to every corner of the globe, and annual rings that were present long before Hippocrates examined his first patient. Those who we teach and are about to teach are Medicine's abundant fruit.

If my recent trip to a college campus was any indication, Medicine's harvest should be bountiful for many years to come. What's more, healthier strains and newer varieties of fruit should continue to appear in the harvest.

Oh, by the way, my son won the essay contest and the scholarship. Like I always say, the fruit doesn't fall far from the tree!

June, 1996

CHOICES

L ife has never been easy for Pete or Jan. Pete had his first myocardial infarction 13 years ago and, today, at the grand old age of 48, he continues to be the victim of an incredible array of disabling illnesses.

Instead of a mid-life crisis, try 3 myocardial infarctions, congestive heart failure, malignant hypertension, emphysema, recurrent nephrolithiasis, cervical and lumbo-sacral disc disease, crippling osteoarthritis, peptic ulcer disease, chronic sinusitis, and a few nervous breakdowns on for size. Pete has, and after multiple cardiac catheterizations, a 5-vessel coronary artery bypass, and numerous sinus surgeries, he can only wonder what it would be like to feel well if only for single day.

Jan has been at Pete's side through all his adversity, and in trying to be a good wife, she has frequently neglected her own health. Lumbo-sacral disc disease, osteoarthritis, assorted radiculopathies, chronic gastritis, and multiple allergies have slowed Jan down, but have not kept her from providing constant emotional support for her husband, from raising their two sons, or from working full-time.

Coping with multiple chronic illnesses has been difficult for Pete and Jan, but not as difficult as trying to pay for their on-going medical care. Pete has already used up his lifetime benefits with one insurer, and even though total disability entitles him to Social Security benefits, he is prohibited from using Medicare as his primary health insurer because of the family major medical coverage that Jan receives at work.

For the past few years, Pete and Jan have been sending all of their medical and surgical bills to Jan's insurer for reimbursement through her major medical coverage. To be sure, major medical payments have taken a bite out of Pete and Jan's medical bills, but deductibles, co-payments, and drug bills have left them in a perpetual state of financial hardship.

In my 13-year association with Pete and Jan, I have billed their insurances for all their health care and have never billed them for any amounts not paid by their insurance companies. Unfortunately, hospitals, laboratories, pharmacies, and a number of other physicians have not been as willing to write off their balances.

Pete and Jan epitomize America's "working poor." Earning too much to qualify for financial aid but not enough to comfortably pay for their health care, they are sadly destined to spend their entire lives a few giant steps behind their overdue bills.

Pete and Jan were in my office today, and to say that they were both depressed is an understatement. When I inquired about their obvious depression, Jan started to cry and handed me a letter from her employer.

Jan's employer is in the process of enrolling his employees in an HMO. The letter informed Jan of her option to pay a nominal fee and receive health care for her entire family from the HMO or to continue her current health care insurance at a monthly cost which would equal an entire week's pay.

The idea of having to pay one week's salary for conventional health insurance brought tears to Jan's eyes. The idea of joining an HMO, and thereby forfeiting the right to medical care by the physician of her choice, made her angry.

As we explore the notion of health care reform, freedom of choice becomes a major consideration. Where health care is concerned, physicians and patients must have freedom of choice because, without such freedom, legitimate health care reform cannot occur.

I do not participate in any HMO programs because HMOs do not provide me with freedom of choice. With HMOs, I am not free to choose my patients, my methods or rates of reimbursement, or my standards of practice.

If Pete and Jan were to join an HMO, they would also be deprived of freedom of choice. They would not be free to choose the physicians of their choice, the quality of their medical care, or even the frequency with which they might be able to obtain medical care.

To most patients, a list of participating HMO physicians is meaningless and, at best, only a spurious example of freedom of choice. So, too, are the various HMO programs that represent little more than rationed health care.

Over the past 13 years, Pete has had many medical and surgical emergencies, and timely medical intervention has allowed him to be a survivor rather than a statistic. Without a concerned primary care physician, who was aware of Pete's many concurrent medical problems, and without an available team of skilled medical and surgical sub-specialists, such timely intervention might not have been possible.

If health care reform can do no better than destroy existing doctor-patient relationships and herd patients into HMOs, managed care, and health care alliances, the entire process would be better left uninitiated. The end result of health care reform should be an improvement of our current health care delivery system and not the short-sighted termination of the many tried and true relationships that have taken many years for Americans to develop with their physicians.

Over the past 13 years, Pete and Jan have convinced me of their gratitude for my professional services. They may not have been able to pay their insurance deductibles or co-payments, but an occasional loaf of zucchini bread or a carrot cake, as well as many sincere words of thanks, have more than covered any outstanding balances.

Considering the rewarding professional relationship I have shared with Pete and Jan, I am not about to abandon them. Accordingly, I have helped them work out a plan that will provide comprehensive health care without leading them into further debt.

For starters, I have advised Jan to enroll in the HMO with her two sons. They will probably never use the HMO for their medical care, but their enrollment will guarantee them hospitalization in the case of any unforeseen emergency.

For their regular medical care, Jan and her two sons will continue to see me. To this end, I have already offered to provide their medical care free of charge.

Insofar as Pete will no longer be covered under Jan's health insurance, he will be able to use Medicare as his primary insurer. I plan to start billing Medicare for Pete's care, and I am sure his other physicians will agree to do the same.

Providing pro bono medical care to Jan and her two sons will do little to bring about health care reform, but it will do a lot to ease the financial burden of a needy family. Not every physician can afford to provide pro bono care to patients, but it is reassuring to know that freedom of choice affords many physicians this luxury.

For physicians, freedom of choice preserves the autonomy of a medical practice and the ability to provide pro bono medical services and other charitable concessions when the need arises. For patients, freedom of choice facilitates competent medical care and guarantees the continuity of such care.

Providing free medical care to Jan and her two sons will probably lower my yearly income by a few hundred bucks, but this dent in my profit structure probably won't stop me from putting bread on the table. If it does, I know where I can get some awfully tasty carrot cake.

August, 1994

TRUE CONFESSIONS

I have a confession to make. I didn't watch the final episode of ***Seinfeld***.

I watch a great deal of television, but I didn't watch the final installment of the popular sitcom. In truth, I didn't watch the first episode of ***Seinfeld*** either—or any other episode for that matter.

While I'm examining my conscience, I should probably also tell you that I still haven't seen the movie, ***Titanic***. Over the years, I've probably seen as many movies as anyone reading this essay, but I still haven't seen the latest cinematic version of the sea epic.

I'll probably see the movie when it hits the video stores or the movie channels on television. ***Rocky*** was the last movie I actually saw in a theater, so I'm used to seeing movies after they've had the chance to age a bit.

There are many other things I could tell you that would probably make you wonder about me. For starters, I've never dined on the Orient Express, gambled in Las Vegas, or spent a single night at a Disney resort.

What's more, I don't golf, I'm not one for social clubs or professional organizations, and I don't hold season tickets issued by any athletic team, opera company, or theater league. I cut my own grass, I do most of my own home and office repairs, and I even take out my own garbage.

While I'm still soul-searching, I also need to tell you that I never worry about cholesterol when I'm enjoying a steak, I enjoy listening to any style of music that is performed well, and I would much rather watch kids playing ball in a sandlot than professionals playing in a modern stadium. Furthermore, I like my whiskey straight, my wine dry, and my beer any way but light.

Finally, you should probably know that I actually enjoy the taste of kielbasi; I truly believe that front-end alignments are a myth; and I actually get a kick out of watching that vaudeville known as heavy-weight wrestling. I'd tell you more, but it's summertime, and I've already exceeded the number of public confessions I usually make during seasons heralded by the return of sunshine to the Northeast.

In my 49 years on this mortal coil, I've developed my own list of likes and dislikes, my own way of doing things, and my own time table. People usually know where I stand, and quite frequently, it's behind the line that separates yours truly from a whole slew of people who firmly embrace the art of thinking conventionally.

When 200-million people have a bad idea, it's still a bad idea. I must confess that I truly enjoy apprising people of that fact.

Now, if you're wondering what all this has to do with managed care, listen up. This treatise doth beseech a moral.

I have never participated in managed care because I am philosophically opposed to any health care delivery system that would ration health care to patients and fees to physicians so that corporate profits might be ensured. In my simple universe, health care is about highly-trained professionals helping sick people and not about an insurance company's current stock price.

I have never participated in managed care, and I must confess that my medical practice has not suffered because of that decision. Not only have 99% of my insured patients stuck with traditional health insurance plans to remain in my practice, but my professional life has been free of the bureaucratic entanglements that have earned managed care its well-deserved notoriety.

By avoiding managed care, I have maintained total control over my medical practice. No one tells me what tests to order, what treatments to render, or what drugs to prescribe.

By avoiding managed care, I have simplified my professional life. Instead of wasting my life resubmitting bills, faxing patient records for review, and listening to irritating telephone music while a managed care secretary prepares to refuse pre-authorization for a test or treatment, I have preserved the time my patients and profession require.

If managed care was everything that government and the insurance industry would have us believe, medical journals would not be teeming with articles about managed care's widespread financial misdirection and regrettable treatment failures. If managed care was any more than just a passing fancy, the same journals would not be laden with the testimonies of physicians who have discovered and rediscovered the joys, feasibility, and advantages of practicing medicine outside the managed care arena.

Insofar as my day is almost finished and I don't have a few hours of managed care paperwork still sitting on my desk, I think I'll fix some Cajun salmon on the barbie. After dinner, I think I'll just sit back and watch a movie or some television.

Tonight may be a good night to go channel surfing and find some reruns of **Seinfeld** to watch. I'd go to the movies to see **Titanic**, but I already know how it ends!

June, 1998

A NEW DOCTOR AND AN
OLD DILEMMA

Newsweek recently published an interesting article by a young physician in residency training. The article chronicled a motor vehicle accident on a country road, the on-site heroics of a physician/ motorist who witnesses the accident, and the accident's aftermath.

This past February, a physician decided to take a break from his residency training and visit the historic battlefield of Gettysburg, Pa. As he was leaving Gettysburg, he was eye-witness to a motor vehicle accident in which a Ford Bronco collided with a small pickup truck.

As the physician and his companion drove past the damaged pickup, they saw the driver's head hanging over the edge of the smashed passenger-side window. The driver was unconscious and cyanotic, his neck was crushed, and his chest slowly heaved against an obstructed airway.

Approaching the truck, the physician could smell alcohol, and clearly see a half-dozen empty beer bottles on the floor of the truck. Sickened by the noisome odor that permeated the truck, the physician instructed a passerby to summon an ambulance, and proceeded to render assistance to the dying truck driver.

With the aid of his companion, the physician carefully moved the driver from the truck's windowsill. Fighting the stench of alcohol, he then tried unsuccessfully to blow air into the cyanotic driver's lungs.

Realizing that he was dealing with an obstructed airway, the young doctor took a large intravenous needle from a medical kit in his car and inserted it into what was left of the accident victim's throat. Air began to immediately whistle through the needle and the victim's life was saved.

An ambulance arrived shortly thereafter and the accident victim was taken to a hospital where he underwent successful throat reconstruction. Less than a week after the surgery, the patient signed himself out of the hospital because of his reported inability to obtain alcoholic beverages in the hospital.

Upon later hearing of the physician's heroics, one of his senior professors told him that he did the right thing medically. He also told the resident that he risked his medical career by attempting to save the accident victim's life.

When the physician asked his professor what he should have done, the professor replied, "Drive on." The professor also told his student that, if the driver had turned out to be a quadriplegic, his rescuer might never have practiced medicine again, thanks to the army of lawyers who would stand in line to get such a case.

Taking his professor's advice into consideration, the physician reflected that, on the day he graduated from medical school, he took an oath to serve the sick and the injured, truly believing that he would be able to do just that. He also admitted that, based on his professor's reaction to the way he responded to a recent emergency, he would simply drive past any future accidents without offering assistance.

There is little question that many physicians understand this young physician's dilemma, and would also look away from any emergency rather than risking a malpractice suit. The reason is obvious.

Once upon a time, physicians, who were found guilty of medical malpractice, were fully backed by their insurance companies and state catastrophic loss funds. Following a malpractice suit, such physicians might have had their malpractice insurance premiums raised or their policies cancelled, but their personal assets were generally not threatened.

Once upon a time, people also had a better understanding of concepts like gratitude and decency. Lawyers weren't as quick to sue Good

Samaritans for malpractice, and accident victims weren't as quick to let them.

The times have changed. Today, multi-million dollar malpractice awards that exceed insurance and catastrophic loss fund coverage can easily wipe out a physician's entire estate or personal fortune.

To add another fly to the ointment, many lawyers are currently testing the legal waters by filing simultaneous civil and criminal charges against physicians in cases of medical malpractice. When a criminal charge of "heinous neglect" is filed against a physician, malpractice insurers could potentially wash their hands of the case, thereby forcing the physician to pay for his or her own defense as well any court awards to the plaintiff.

With financial ruin and criminal charges as potential consequences, it is easy to understand why an ever-increasing number of physicians are vowing not to play the role of Good Samaritan. What is not as easy to understand is where this lunacy will finally end.

If physicians drive past accidents today, what will they do tomorrow? Will they run and hide every time they see a customer choking in a restaurant, or a child knocked unconscious at a little league game, or a patient about to experience a cardiac arrest in a hospital ward?

And what will the courts of the future have to say about a physician who gets caught running away from an emergency? Will the courts view the medical negligence of a physician who stops at the scene of an accident as harshly as the criminal negligence of a physician who fails to stop?

The first paragraph in the Eighth Edition of ***Harrison's Principles Of Internal Medicine*** reads as follows: "No greater opportunity, responsibility, or obligation is given to an individual than that of serving as a physician. In treating the suffering, there is need for technical skill, scientific knowledge, and human understanding. The person who uses these with courage, with humility, and with wisdom will provide a unique service and will build an enduring edifice of character. The physician should ask of destiny no more than this and be content with no less."

What follows in Harrison's textbook are 2,008 pages of instructions on how to diagnose and treat human illness. Without a complete understanding of the book's first paragraph, however—without a complete understanding of a physician's purpose, mastery of the ensuing pages would appear to be little more than a futile academic exercise.

As physicians, we are distinguished from all other people by our ability to intervene in human suffering. To run away from an emergency is to thoughtlessly renounce the very privilege that makes our profession unique and, yes, special.

If I had been this young resident's advisor, and learned about his afternoon in Gettysburg, I would have congratulated him on a job well done. I would have also encouraged him to share his story and his fears with the news media, legislators, and representatives of such politically-oriented organizations as the American Medical Association.

I would have challenged him to use his experience to the best advantage of his profession. I would have challenged him to fight for malpractice reform and for the right of a Good Samaritan to render competent emergency medical care without fear of malpractice litigation.

Above all else, I would have urged this doctor to continue to follow the same instincts that allowed him to save the life of a human being. That life may have belonged to a troubled man with an alcohol problem, but it could have just as easily belonged to someone else.

That life could have belonged to someone's father, or fiancée, or best friend. It could have belonged to someone who had the power to enact the kind of legislative reform that the medical profession so desperately needs.

As an advisor, I would have cautioned the doctor about society's pitfalls. As a fellow-physician, I would have cautioned him about the limitations of his profession.

As a human being, I would have cautioned him about many other things. Given the premise of an accident on a country road near Gettysburg, however, I would never have cautioned him to "Drive on."

June, 1995

A DEJA POINT OF VU

L egend has it that Yogi Berra was once awakened in the middle of the night by an unexpected phone call. A New York Yankee teammate called to tell Yogi that he had just won the American League's "Most Valuable Player" award.

After he offered the appropriate congratulations, the teammate apologized for disturbing Berra's sleep. "That's alright," Yogi replied, "I had to get up to answer the phone anyway!"

In addition to being remembered as one of the greatest catchers in baseball history, Yogi Berra has also become famous for his unique command of the English language. The Hall-of-Famer is credited with describing a close game as "a real cliff dweller," informing a business office that they misspelled his name when they issued a check worded, "Pay To Bearer," and coining the phrase, "it's like *deja vu* all over again."

If you've been following the news media's coverage of doctors' unions over the past few months, you've probably come to the conclusion that many writers and reporters have also started taking liberties with the English language. Their various and sundry reports on the American Medical Association's planned development of national labor organizations have left many Americans with confusion over what constitutes a union, and with the false impression that the entire medical profession has finally decided to unionize.

For the record, the AMA voted this past June to develop, not a doctors' union, but various affiliated national labor organizations that would allow only those physicians employed by hospitals, insurers, or the government to engage in collective bargaining with their employers. These labor organizations, which would also represent certain groups of physicians-in-training, would potentially affect only one in seven American physicians.

Despite news media assertions to the contrary, the AMA did not vote to form a doctors' union in June. In fact, AMA trustees were even reluctant to authorize the formation of a limited labor organization for employed physicians, but ultimately decided to honor the wishes of the AMA's House of Delegates and endorse the proposal.

The leadership of the AMA is philosophically opposed to the notion of physicians belonging to a traditional labor union. The AMA leaders see significant downside potential in endorsing physician unionization because of potential harm to the AMA's image, membership, and finances.

However, with Governor Bush already signing a law allowing Texas physicians to engage in collective bargaining, and the Campbell Bill, which would ensure collective bargaining rights for all American physicians, making headway in Congress, the AMA leadership had little alternative but to hop on the running boards of the physicians' labor bandwagon. The resulting endorsement of physician labor organizations by the AMA has been interpreted by many analysts as little more than a symbolic gesture.

In response to the recent actions by the AMA, many physicians have published articles and editorials supporting full-scale unionization of the American medical profession. Most of these writers have cited the need for collective bargaining with managed care as the major reason for physicians to unionize.

Although collective bargaining with managed care is a valid reason for unionization, there are many other valid reasons. For starters, unionization would set the stage for the professional standardization of health care in America.

Unionization would help ensure physician competence by allowing new guidelines for graduate and continuing medical education to be established. It would foster the implementation of independent and unbiased peer review activities, as well as the development of efficient arbitration programs within the courts.

Unionization would provide physicians with many badly needed services. It would standardize physicians' fees; create group purchasing networks; assist in physician placement; develop affordable malpractice, health, disability, and life insurance programs for physicians and their families; provide its members with a wide range of financial services; and create programs for rehabilitating impaired physicians and modifying the careers of disabled physicians.

Unionization would allow physicians to determine, rather than follow, the course of health care in America. It would allow the medical profession to become more active politically, assume a greater roll in the electoral process, and finally create a level playing field for dealings with industry, the courts, and our legislatures.

Unionization would allow physicians to be helped by professional representatives in disputes with licensing boards, hospitals, and insurers. It would provide physicians with the help they needed to guarantee smoke-free public facilities, drug-free schools, and pollution-free environments in their communities.

Unionization would do much more than just ensure collective bargaining with managed care. Significantly, unionization would empower the American medical profession to prevent mistakes like managed care from ever happening again.

The AMA has been reluctant to call for the unionization of the American medical profession, and for this much, physicians should be grateful. The AMA is, has always been, and most likely, will always be a medical society incapable of generating the kind of dynamic force necessary to affect positive social, political, or professional change.

A physicians' union developed by the AMA would be little more than an expanded version of the current AMA. To paraphrase a former Yankee great, it would be little more than more of the same.

The American medical profession needs to form a union unencumbered by any ties to the AMA. To meet new challenges, the American medical profession needs a new identity.

As a child, I loved watching Yankee greats like Yogi Berra, Mickey Mantle, Roger Maris, Bobby Richardson, Tony Kubek, Whitey Ford, and Moose Skowron win one championship after another. Even in my youth, I appreciated the value of teamwork and unity.

Today, I continue to value teamwork and unity, and clearly see how such attributes would enhance the medical profession and help create a health care delivery system that was run by health care professionals rather than politicians and business executives. Just like the Yankee teams of old, a union of American physicians would set new standards and be a winner on everybody's scorecard.

In an age of too many pressing health care issues, a physicians' union might be all that it takes to return medicine to its rightful owners, namely America's skilled and dedicated physicians and the millions of patients who have been entrusted to our care. Then, you might say, it would be like *deja vu* all over again!

September, 1999

THE OPTION TO LIVE

For the past two years, June's home has been the first stop on my weekly round of house calls. Before she became home-bound, the forty year-old woman had been admitted to a major medical center for the diagnosis and treatment of metastatic lung cancer.

Throughout her prolonged hospitalization, June endured multiple invasive procedures, as well as attempts at chemotherapy and radiation therapy. Her hospital course was as much a nightmare for June as being told that lung cancer was metastasizing through her entire body.

Somehow, June managed to survive her hospitalization, and she returned home after being told that nothing else could be done for her at the world-renowned medical center. June doesn't remember the details of the final meeting with her attending physician, but she vividly remembers overhearing him tell a group of medical students and residents that there was nothing left for her to do but go home and die.

Prior to being discharged from the hospital, June's attending physician arranged for her to receive home health services from a large agency. June named me as her private physician, and prior to the start of her home nursing care, the director of the agency called to acquaint me with her agency's services.

Following a few pleasantries, the director informed me that I would receive periodic updates on June's progress from her agency. She also informed me that I would be asked to sign recertification forms on occasion and write certain prescriptions.

When I began to ask the director a few specific questions about June's home nursing care, she told me not to worry because her agency employed a number of consulting physicians who would provide June's nurses with information and instructions. Although none of these physicians would ever visit June at home, I was assured that they would handle her problems over the phone and serve as her attending physicians whenever she required hospitalization.

The director's brief introduction to her agency's services made me quickly realize that, even though I was June's personal physician, I was being taken out of the loop that would be responsible for June's future health care. I didn't like the plan, and even more importantly, neither did June or her family.

Following a major redefinition of roles, I agreed to visit June at home on a weekly basis, and the home health agency agreed to follow my care plan. For the past two years, the relationship has been beneficial to everyone concerned, and it has allowed June to remain at home where she continues to comfortably survive a terminal illness.

With the need for health care reform so urgent a matter in the United States, the development of economical and efficient home health care programs is taking on added importance. If how to take care of more chronically and terminally ill patients with fewer health care dollars is the question, home health care is undeniably the answer.

Many of today's home health care programs fall short of providing optimal services to their patients because they involve physicians in only a peripheral manner. Patients are generally grateful for competent nursing care, but they also have a frequently unfulfilled need to regularly see their physician.

Studies have shown that patients with chronic or terminal illnesses who see a physician regularly survive significantly longer than patients with similar illnesses who do not see a physician on a regular basis. There is very little that can replace physician expertise in the management of serious illness.

Obviously, not every physician has the ability to make house calls, but many more physicians would consider the practice under the right circumstances. House calls don't have to be time-consuming "afternoon tea and photo album sessions," but can be conducted with the same efficiency as hospital or office visits.

Many physicians object to making house calls because of the travel time and poor third party reimbursement. Not much can be done about travel time, but physicians could certainly be given a financial incentive to make house calls.

A few years ago, Canada solved its hospital overutilization problem by paying physicians more to treat patients in offices than in hospitals. In a short period of time, the census in many Canadian hospitals dropped from 90% to 50%, clearly demonstrating the role of financial incentives in health care.

A similar approach could be taken in the United States. Physicians could be paid higher rates to make house calls than to treat patients in hospitals or skilled nursing facilities.

Travel allowances could also be made. The end result would be a dramatic reduction in the overall cost of treating chronically or terminally ill patients.

There is little question that most chronically ill patients would rather be at home than in a hospital or some other extended care facility. With each hospitalization or institutionalization, patients risk nosocomial infections, mental status changes, and unforeseen injury.

Not every patient is fortunate enough to be able to receive medical care in their own home. Those who do receive home health care, however, generally do so in greater comfort and with greater safety than patients who are hospitalized.

As a representative of Medicine's new breed of physicians, I derive a great deal of personal satisfaction from being an old-fashioned country doctor who still makes house calls. If it is true that "what goes around, comes around," many other physicians are about to discover the many advantages of making house calls, and this discovery should be encouraged and facilitated by home health care services, third-party payers, and those involved in health care reform.

In too many cases, the role of the physician in home health care has been reduced to signing order sheets and recertification forms. My experience with June has proven that a physician's role in home health care can be a great deal more.

Two years ago, a technologically-advanced medical center sent June home to die. In the interim, a loving family, a dedicated group of nurses, and an old-fashioned country doctor have given June another option—the option to live.

April, 1994

SEARCHING FOR PERFECTION

A beautiful story is currently making its way across the internet. It is the story of a loving and insightful father, his learning-disabled son, and an age-old question.

During a recent parent-teacher meeting at a school for children with learning disabilities, a parent observed that the very existence of children with disabilities, handicaps, and serious illnesses negated the premise of a perfect God. In response, another parent told the following story.

While walking through a park, the parent and his young son came upon a group of boys playing baseball. The father watched as a smile came to the face of his son who loved baseball but never played the game because of various disabilities.

As he watched his son look with envy at the boys who were playing the game, the father decided to help his son take a giant step forward. Approaching the apparent leader of one of the teams, the father asked if his son would be able to join the game.

"Mister, our team is getting killed," the young team captain said, "and I'm sure your son can't play any worse than we've been playing all day. There's only one inning left, but your son can finish the game on our team if he wants."

Making no attempts at containing the joy he was feeling, the proud father applauded as his awkward son picked up a glove and ran out to the outfield. As the father shouted encouragement from the sidelines, the players watched as their newest teammate struggled to overcome his obvious spasticity en route to his position in the field.

For reasons that no one understood, their new teammate's presence in the field seemed to inspire the other players to play harder. Unlike previous innings, the team was able to hold their opponents scoreless and return to the bench for their final turn at bat.

Down by more runs than they cared to remember, the team continued to be inspired by their new teammate, and each player seemed to step up to the plate with greater confidence and greater purpose. Hits quickly turned into runs, and by the time the dust had settled, the bases were loaded and the potential winning run—the team's newest and most inexperienced player, was about to step up to the plate.

The father was certain that the team would not allow his son to bat with two outs and the game on the line, but much to his surprise, his son picked up a bat and approached home plate. When it became obvious that the youngster didn't know how to hold a bat or where to stand in the batter's box, the team captain called a timeout, and following some quick instructions and encouragement, the young boy prepared to bat for the first time in his life.

Realizing that the would-be hitter was out of his league in more ways than one, the pitcher, who was also touched by his disabled opponent's participation in the game, moved closer to home plate, and instead of throwing the ball hard and fast, merely lobbed the ball toward the batter. Despite the pitcher's best intentions, the batter swung late and missed the pitch by a wide margin.

Having carefully observed the batter's awkward swing, the pitcher moved even closer toward home plate and delivered the next pitch underhanded as if to hit his unskilled opponent's bat. Despite a late and clumsy swing, the perfect placement of the pitch allowed the batter to hit the ball on the ground back to the pitcher.

Still stunned by the fact that he had successfully hit a baseball, the youngster had to be prompted by his father and teammates to run to first base. As he started to run, the pitcher picked up the baseball, but instead of easily throwing it to first base for the final out, he threw the ball deep into right field.

As the other runners made their way around the bases, their newest teammate finally arrived at first base, and following more prompting by the first baseman, started running toward second. Upon arriving at second, he was quickly turned in the direction of third base by the opposing team's shortstop.

Instead of throwing the ball to third base for an easy out, the right fielder threw the ball far over the third baseman's head. Rather than attempting to retrieve the ball, the third baseman turned the exhausted but excited runner toward home plate.

With his heart pounding, a very proud father watched his son cross home plate with the winning run. Through tearful eyes, he watched as his son was mobbed by his teammates and given a hero's reception.

The father told this story at the parent-teacher meeting to demonstrate that God's perfection can be seen even when such apparent imperfections as disabilities, handicaps, and illnesses abound. "My son, imperfect though he may appear to some, was an important part of a perfect plan because he was able to bring out God's perfection in all the other players from both teams," the father told his audience.

As physicians, we have witnessed the imperfection of disease, suffering, and infirmity. Most of us have wondered and tried futilely to explain how a perfect God could create such imperfection.

"How did God let this happen?" we have heard patients ask. "How could God let this happen?" we have asked ourselves.

Just as a disabled child was able to inspire God's perfection on a baseball field, sick and suffering patients inspire God's perfection in medical offices, clinics, and hospitals. God's perfection can be seen in the process of healing, a process that has been entrusted to those of us who have dedicated our lives to the practice of medicine.

In a world of managed care profiteering, frivolous malpractice litigation, and the ongoing socialization of medicine, it is easy to lose sight of who we are. Some would have us be health care managers or participating providers, but those of us who call ourselves doctors or physicians are healers.

We live in a world where perfection is not always apparent, but as physicians, we have been blessed with the opportunity to participate in a miraculous process that heals, restores, and sometimes even perfects. We are healers, and no less than the father who watched his son being carried off the field on the shoulders of his teammates, we should swell with pride over the importance of the role we have been chosen to play and the perfect plan that made such a role possible.

June, 2000

A CERTAIN SMILE

For 81 years, the one constant in her life was a smile. She smiled when things were good, and during the many years she was confined to a bed, she smiled as if to hint that things could be better.

A massive intra-cranial hemorrhage took away her speech, her ability to swallow, and her ability to walk. The one thing that it didn't take away was her smile.

To some degree, her smile made it easier for her daughter to abandon any semblance of a normal life and assume total responsibility for an ailing mother's care. Her smile also made it easier for her son-in-law to turn his home into a veritable skilled nursing facility, and make caring for her a top priority.

I know that her smile made it easier for me to make the many house calls that were needed to treat her seemingly endless array of aspiration pneumonias, bouts of painful osteoarthritis, and multiple gastrointestinal maladies. I'm sure that most of the nurses and therapists I sent to aid in her care would say the same.

A few weeks before Christmas, the smile was coaxed from her face by pain from a severely ulcerated tongue. From the very outset, I knew that she would continue to experience pain until the diseased teeth that caused her tongue ulcerations were extracted, but I also knew that getting her into a dentist's office or hospital for surgical intervention would be no small task.

Fortunately, I have a friend who is a talented dentist and acquaintance of my patient and her family. When I called and explained the dilemma, he immediately offered his assistance.

A few days later, he gave up a free afternoon to accompany me on a memorable house call. The cost of disposable materials was $5, and the cost of injectable drugs was $10, but the sight of a dentist and internist combining forces to relieve pain and restore an elderly patient's smile in the comfort of her own home was priceless!

If for no other reason than the muscle activity involved, it is much easier to smile than frown. Similarly, it is much easier to be kind, charitable, and helpful than mean, selfish, or spiteful.

Being kind to another person is a defining characteristic of our human nature. Being unkind is much more difficult because, unlike kindness which is generally spontaneous, unkindness must be planned and executed which frequently makes it difficult.

Life events can create malevolence in even the kindest people, but ill will is a learned trait that can be modified. Most people want to be kind to others but frequently need to be encouraged to express kindness to its fullest extent.

Many talented professionals also want to stretch the envelope of their kindness and reach out to greater numbers of people in ways that might put their many skills to better use. Many are willing to be accessible, charitable, and even unconventional for little more than a sincere request and modicum of gratitude.

For the past few months, my patient was seldom seen without a smile. A few days ago, however, her smile proved more enduring than the rest of her frail body.

At her funeral, a number of people commented that she seemed to have died with a smile on her face. To those of us who labored to restore and maintain it, that certain smile will always have special meaning.

March, 2001

GETTING PLASTERED

For the past few days, I've been getting plastered. It sounds like I've been on a drunken binge but, in reality, I've been watching my office ceilings being repaired.

In the process, I've seen plaster speckle my rugs, furniture, and even a few moving targets. I was about to suggest a skin biopsy to one of my elderly patients before I realized that a small dollop of plaster had silently fallen on her neck and dried into the exact configuration of a seborrheic keratosis!

For the past few days, my office has looked more like a battle zone than a rural medical clinic. Like I said, I've been getting plastered.

Larry is the plastermeister who is responsible for my office's current disarray. He's actually a good plasterer, but he's prone to talking and gesticulating while he works, which explains a great deal of the mess.

Larry's been around this area for quite some time, and he knows the bottom line on just about everybody. In fact, this morning he started reminiscing about his old friend, Doctor Sam.

Sam was once a prominent general practitioner in this area. Unfortunately, a few misunderstandings snow-balled into a larger-than-life dilemma, and Sam was forced to close his practice.

The whole mess started when Sam was joined in a malpractice suit against a small rural hospital. The suit was of the "nickel/dime" variety, but it created a major rift between Sam and his hospital.

The hospital tried to blame Sam for the patient's alleged injury, and Sam maintained that the hospital was at fault. The end result was that the patient's lawyer got a cruise out of the deal, the patient got a cup of coffee, and Sam and his hospital became bitter enemies.

One thing led to another and the hospital started picking on Sam for delinquent charts, utilization problems, and even tardiness at medical staff meetings. Sam got into a perpetual tug-of-war with the hospital's medical director, and before long, he found his admitting privileges being suspended for trivial reasons.

Stories about Sam's on-going battle with the hospital were quickly transformed into fairy tales in which Sam was depicted as some kind of ogre. In a very short time, Sam's practice and reputation were irreparably damaged.

Sam was closing his medical practice at the same time I was opening mine. Although I never met Sam, I heard him criticized by a number of different physicians, including a few who never met him.

Sam had reached the summit of his profession only to fall into an endless chasm of disgrace. Sam had saved the lives of many patients and nurtured the careers of many young physicians but, in retrospect, very few people had anything positive to say about the man.

When I told Larry that I never met Sam, he smiled and started recounting his experiences with the physician.

"I'm here today because of Doctor Sam," Larry said. "Years ago, he removed a lump from under my arm. It was melanoma, and it was all through my body. He sent me to a cancer specialist, who told me that I was too far gone for any treatment. The cancer specialist also said some nasty things about Doctor Sam. I could never understand how he could criticize Doctor Sam when he never met the man."

Larry paused and tears started to come to his eyes.

"I went back to Doctor Sam and he started making long-distance phone calls all around the country," Larry said. "He finally got me into a special program in Maryland. I went down there once a week for quite a few months and got some kind of experimental chemotherapy. The treatment worked, and I've been cured for over ten years. There were twenty-five of us in that experimental program and only two of us are still alive"

Larry paused and wiped his eyes, plastering his cheeks in the process.

"I had to stop working for a while because of the melanoma," Larry continued. "You know that Doctor Sam kept taking care of me and my family for free. He got into some trouble a few years ago, and he had to move. I never got his new address, and I'm sorry I didn't. I've been meaning to send him a Christmas card, and thank him for all he did for me and my family."

I don't know if Sam was more a saint or sinner, but I do know that unfair accusations and false rumors have closed many medical practices and ended many medical careers. I also know that the medical profession is fraught with physicians who, because of arrogance, insecurity, or any of a number of other personal shortcomings, seem to make a habit of openly criticizing their colleagues without sufficient reason.

Constructive criticism is one thing but uninformed oral fibrillation is quite another. The former can save a career while the latter has prematurely ended the careers of many innocent physicians.

My years in the medical profession have left me with the belief that very few physicians are as good as they claim to be, and very few physicians are as bad as others would have them be. My years have also taught me that it is easier to completely remove dry plaster from a new rug than it is to restore the good name of someone who has been the target of unjust public criticism.

To this day, many physicians still go out of their way to criticize Sam. On the flip side, Larry still praises Sam as the competent physician and caring friend who saved his life.

Perhaps the philosopher, Charles Sanders Pierce, was thinking of someone like Sam when he wrote, "Full many a gem of purest ray serene the dark, unfathomed caves of ocean bear; full many a flower is born to blush unseen, and waste its sweetness on the desert air."

November, 1994

THE ERRATA OF MY WAYS

Recognized as the founder of American pragmatism, Charles Sanders Peirce was born in Cambridge, Massachusetts in 1839. Schooled in mathematics and physics at Harvard University, he taught logic at Johns Hopkins before becoming a physicist for the U.S. Coastal and Geodetic Survey.

He retired in 1890 and devoted the last 24 years of his life to philosophy. In 1878, *Popular Science Monthly* published Peirce's paper, *"How To Make Our Ideas Clear."*

In this paper, Peirce wrote, "But I may be asked what I have to say to all the minute facts of history, forgotten never to be recovered, to the lost books of the ancients, to the buried secrets. Full many a gem of purest ray serene, the dark unfathomed caves of ocean bear; full many a flower is born to blush unseen, and waste its sweetness on the desert air."

Nowhere in his paper did Peirce quote any other authors. Nowhere did he give the reader any reason to believe that the passages contained therein were written by anyone other than Peirce himself.

In an article recently published in the medical literature, I quoted the preceding passage and credited it to Charles Sanders Peirce. A number of readers have since argued that the passage was not written by Peirce but by Thomas Gray in his *Elegy Written In A Country Churchyard*.

On researching the matter, I discovered that Gray had indeed written about flowers being born to blush unseen in the mid-1700's, a full century before the same words were written by Peirce. I also rediscovered that it was not uncommon for writers of the 18th and 19th centuries to incorporate previously-written passages into their books and papers without quoting or otherwise giving formal credit to the original authors of the borrowed passages.

Ergo, the passage in question must be credited to Thomas Gray. However, anyone who has ever read **How To Make Our Ideas Clear** but not **Elegy Written In A Country Churchyard** would have little reason to attribute the passage to anyone but Charles Sanders Peirce.

So, am I to bear the slings and arrows of outrageous fortune for accurately quoting a renowned philosopher who forgot to mention that his best lines were borrowed from an elegy by an esteemed poet? Am I to suffer injustice for justice sake just so that I may stand corrected?

Verily, verily, I say unto thee that what appears Gray to one man is Peirce to another. Fret not, however, for this treatise doth beseech a moral.

In Medicine, most of us have been taught by the "see one, do one, teach one" method. We were schooled in the art of practicing what we learned and teaching what we practiced.

Unfortunately, this method is not without fault. As one astute physician observed, "Half of what they teach in medical school is wrong. The trick is to figure out which half is right."

Today, more than ever before, physicians are expected to keep up with Medicine's ever-expanding body of knowledge. To accomplish this, however, physicians have been forced to delegate much of their information-gathering and processing responsibilities to others.

Physicians have been forced to rely on politicians for the latest word on health care reform, the news media for the inside story on the health care industry, and drug reps for the most current information on medical therapy. Physicians have been forced to obtain medical information from individuals outside the medical profession.

We profess what we think we know. Unfortunately, what we think we know is not always what we need to know.

Political lies, sensationalized journalistic fabrications, and bogus medical research have deprived physicians of many a truth. Unfortunately, physicians have all too frequently been the last to know.

As a result, physicians have unwittingly professed half-truths and complete falsehoods to trusting patients who rely on the medical profession for their health and well-being. Patients have suffered the ill consequences, physicians have lost respect, and the special interest groups have profited from deception.

If something sounds too good to be true, it probably is. It behooves all of us in the medical profession to be wary of the plans and products that sound too good to be true, as well as the cheap shots that the same special interest groups employ to achieve opposite, but equally useful, effects.

As physicians, we have a responsibility to our patients and our profession to carefully weigh each modicum of new information before we accept it as being true and worthy of dissemination. We also have a responsibility to our colleagues to openly express our concerns about political plans, medical news, and therapies that leave us with more unanswered questions than definitive answers.

There are many fine medical journals that take pleasure in publishing the concerns of their readers. These journals are the appropriate forum where medical discussions can and should take place.

If a physician is bothered about the direction of health care reform, a new scientific study, or one of Medicine's many current controversies, the appropriate concerns should be shared with the rest of the medical profession. Something a physician writes may prove useful to many grateful colleagues.

If a physician is bothered by something in print, that physician should make his or her objections known. Any journal or journalist worth their sodium chloride should be able to handle an opposing opinion or a therapeutic dose of constructive criticism.

One of the many purposes of communicating in the written form is to inspire the kind of dialogue that will promote both truth and understanding. Having an incorrect belief or assumption corrected promotes both truth and understanding, but neither can be promoted without open communication.

The medical profession is currently being challenged from every conceivable direction by an unprecedented number of external forces. To meet this challenge, physicians must be able to applaud each other's accomplishments and help each other understand that an occasional mistake comes with the territory.

In the movie, **Bull Durham**, Crash Davis hits a homerun that sets a new minor league record. Unfortunately, Crash is the only one in the entire stadium who is aware of the accomplishment.

Commenting on this unusual situation, his girlfriend, Annie Savoy, says, "'Full many a flower is born to blush unseen, and waste its sweetness on the desert air.' Thomas Gray. Or William Cullen Bryant. I don't know—I get them mixed up!"

Thanks, Annie. I'm glad I'm not the only one!

April, 1995

THE OATH OF HIPPOCRATES

I f you are like many physicians, your first exposure to the Hippocratic Oath probably came during your medical school graduation ceremonies. If you are like many other physicians, the Oath you recited during your commencement exercises was probably an abbreviated version of the Hippocratic Oath rather than the original.

Such abbreviated versions have generally allowed physicians to vow that they "will refrain from that which is illegal." However, these same versions have not required physicians to pledge their abstinence from any specific activities.

After my article dealing with the Hippocratic Oath was published in the medical literature a year ago, I received an incredible number of letters from physicians who closely followed the teachings of the Oath, as well as a few letters from physicians who had never read the Hippocratic Oath in its entirety. A number of physicians in this latter group reported being unable to find copies of the Hippocratic Oath even in medical school libraries.

Over the past few decades, the medical profession has become divided on the question of the contemporary relevance of the Hippocratic Oath. Opponents of the Oath have protested that it is an anachronism that has more historical significance than practical importance, while proponents of the Oath have argued that it represents ageless wisdom and is as relevant and applicable today as it was when it was written.

To get a better idea of why this historic document has created so much controversy, consider, if you will, the Oath of Hippocrates. It reads as follows:

"I swear by Apollo the physician, and Æsculapius, and Health, and All-heal, and all the gods and goddesses, that, according to my ability and judgment, I will keep this Oath and stipulations—to reckon him who taught me this Art equally dear to me as my parents, to share my substance with him, and relieve his necessities if required; to look upon his offspring in the same footing as my own brothers, and to teach them this art, if they shall wish to learn it, without fee or stipulation; and that by precept, lecture, and every other mode of instruction, I will impart a knowledge of the Art to my own sons, and those of my teachers, and to disciples bound by a stipulation and oath according to the law of medicine, but to none others. I will follow that system of regimen which, according to my ability and judgment, I consider for the benefit of my patients, and abstain from whatever is deleterious and mischievous. I will give no deadly medicine to any one if asked, nor suggest any such counsel; and in like manner I will not give to a woman a pessary to produce abortion. With purity and with holiness I will pass my life and practice my Art. I will not cut persons laboring under the stone, but will leave this to be done by men who are practitioners of this work. Into whatever houses I enter, I will go into them for the benefit of the sick, and will abstain from every voluntary act of mischief and corruption; and, further, from the seduction of females or males, of freemen and slaves. Whatever, in connection with my professional practice or not, in connection with it, I see or hear, in the life of men, which ought not to be spoken of abroad, I will not divulge, as reckoning that all such should be kept secret. While I continue to keep this Oath unviolated, may it be granted to me to enjoy life and the practice of the art, respected by all men, in all times! But should I trespass and violate this Oath, may the reverse be my lot!"

It would appear that the Hippocratic Oath clearly prohibits physicians from performing abortions, from assisting in suicides, and from participating in a number of other activities that have gained silent acceptance by the medical profession. It would also appear that the Oath clearly prescribes an ethical standard for physicians that set medical practitioners apart from all other professionals.

It can be argued that the medical profession has outgrown the Hippocratic Oath, but it can also be argued that many members of the medical profession have lost sight of a physician's true role in society. In trying to become all things to all people, we may have lost sight of the simplicity involved in coming to the aid of another human being.

As the medical profession continues to experience an unprecedented number of internal and external problems, it may be appropriate for all of us to take time out to redefine the role of the physician in society. A good starting point may be the Hippocratic Oath.

If we give it a chance, the Oath may help us answer some of our profession's most difficult questions. If we continue to hide it from new generations of physicians, the Oath may start to sound more and more like Greek.

January, 1993

MATTERS CONTAGIOUS

A few decades ago, zoo officials decided to destroy one of their facility's most popular attractions, a large gorilla. The animal had developed crippling rheumatoid arthritis, and despite heroic attempts by a team of veterinarians, the gorilla's constant pain could not be brought under control.

Hearing about the zoo's plans to destroy the arthritic gorilla, a medical doctor offered his assistance. The concerned practitioner had a theory about rheumatoid arthritis actually being an infection caused by a species of *streptococcus* and, as such, treatable with antibiotics.

Intrigued by the physician's theory, the zoo officials allowed the practitioner to treat the ailing gorilla with tetracycline. Within a very short period of time, the gorilla's rheumatoid arthritis went into remission, and plans to destroy the animal were canceled.

When I shared this story with a number of different rheumatologists, I was given all sorts of compelling reasons why rheumatoid arthritis could not and should not be misconstrued as the end-result of exposure to *streptococcus.* Despite the skepticism of the rheumatologists, I still wondered if there wasn't a lesson to be learned from an arthritic gorilla.

Following this episode, I closely observed what happened to patients with rheumatoid arthritis who were placed on tetracycline or erythromycin for upper respiratory tract infections. Uniformly, these patients all seemed to experience a small but perceptible decrease in arthritic pain, morning stiffness, and joint immobility while they were taking the antibiotics and a slight exacerbation of these symptoms shortly after the antibiotics were discontinued.

A few months ago, the apparent remission of rheumatoid arthritis in patients treated with minocycline was reported in the scientific literature. An experiment that was disregarded for lack of scientific substance two decades ago has now been reproduced and suddenly shown greater interest by the scientific community.

Without doubt, the scientific community's renewed interest in the cause-and-effect relationship between infection and chronic disease has been fostered by the discovery that peptic ulcers can be caused by the bacteria, **Helicobacter pylori,** and eradicated by a number of conventional antibiotics to which the bacteria has shown sensitivity. This discovery has dramatically changed the way peptic ulcer disease is treated and given the medical profession greater control over a potentially menacing illness.

At the same time that a well-meaning physician was treating a gorilla's rheumatoid arthritis with tetracycline, other physicians were arguing over the value of titrating antacid doses according to gastric pH measurements and the necessity of obtaining weekly blood counts on patients who were taking a new ulcer medication, cimetidine. No one was talking about the possibility of treating peptic ulcers with antibiotics.

Today, of course, talk of treating a greater number of chronic illnesses as infections are becoming more prevalent in medical circles. Who would have thought twenty years ago that medical researchers would one day actually explore the possibility of myocardial infarctions being caused by the bacteria, **Chlamydia pneumoniae?**

And who would have thought twenty years ago that Alzheimer's disease might be the end result of an infectious process? Who would have thought that researchers would one day be able to induce neurologic abnormalities in laboratory animals by injecting them with white blood cells taken from close contacts of patients with Alzheimer's disease?

Who would have thought that researchers would one day postulate that Alzheimer's disease might be caused by the human-to-human transmission of a slow virus, as in the case of other dementing illnesses, such as kuru and Creutzfeldt-Jakob disease? Who would have thought that the world might one day be forced to deal with the ominous reality of contagious dementia?

We are living during an exciting period in Medicine's illustrious history. We are discovering new causes for old diseases and quick fixes for illnesses that were once thought incurable.

We are living at a time when respected scientists are actually starting to talk about heart attacks, arthritis, and dementia being contagious. We are living at a time when a greater number of correct answers are inspiring a greater number of previously unasked questions.

Who is to say that diabetes mellitus, multiple sclerosis, or certain types of cancer won't be the next diseases to be matched with a microorganism and eradicated with an antibiotic? Who is to say that a daily prophylactic dose of an antibiotic won't one day replace aspirin as a means of preventing myocardial infarctions, cerebro-vascular accidents, and who knows what else?

Those of us who are currently practicing medicine are doing so at an incredibly exciting time. We are all helping to create chapters in medical texts that have yet to be written.

This being the case, it would appear that we all have a responsibility to preserve the practice of medicine—a practice that most of us still cherish. We also have a responsibility to protect our profession from the many forces in society that would interfere with our work, stunt our growth, or trespass within our exclusive domain.

Medical research, medical education, and medical practice must be preserved and protected at all costs. They must be preserved and protected for future generations of physicians and patients in the same fashion that they were preserved and protected for all of us.

As current research would suggest, the physicians of tomorrow will undoubtedly be treating a greater number of diseases as infections. Hopefully the same values, attitudes, and principles that have guided generations of physicians will be successfully passed on to our next generation of caregivers, and prove to be as contagious as the diseases these doctors hope to cure.

December, 1997

MEDICAL ERRORS

I n the middle of a heated battle, three atheists sought refuge in a fox-hole.

"Guys, I don't think we're going to survive this mess," the first soldier said.

"You're probably right," the second soldier replied. "Do you think we should say some kind of prayer just in case we've been wrong about things and there is a God somewhere?"

"We probably should," the first soldier agreed, "but I don't know any prayers."

"Me neither," the second soldier said.

"Guys, I used to live across the street from a Catholic church," the third soldier offered, "and in the summertime, when the church windows were open, I used to hear them praying."

"Do you remember how the prayer went?" the first soldier asked.

Folding his hands and looking toward heaven, the third soldier solemnly prayed, "On the B—14; on the N—42!"

The Institute of Medicine's recent report, "To Err Is Human—Building a Safer Health System," has supplied the necessary ammunition for government officials, legislators, lawyers, consumer protection advocates, and various and sundry other watchdogs to start demanding programs that will force physicians and other health care providers to practice safer medicine. The vested interests and political agendas of these individuals and groups notwithstanding, their concerted demand for an immediate and dramatic reduction in the number of medical errors is unequivocal.

The Institute of Medicine is not sure if 44,000 patients die yearly in the United States because of medical errors, or if the number more closely approximates 98,000. Although the study's statistics are grossly inflated, if not bogus, because of wholesale extrapolation, the report does raise an important point.

Pure and simple, too many patients die in the United States each year because of careless errors that could and should have been prevented. The exact number of yearly patient deaths attributable to medical errors is moot, but open to considerably less debate is the fact that a single patient death caused by a preventable error is, was, and will always be one death too many.

The Institute of Medicine's recent study, and more importantly, the reaction of the previously named groups and the American public to that report, is destined to perpetuate the ongoing witch hunt through the rank and file of the American medical profession. Programs that mandate the reporting of medical errors to government or private agencies will invariably lead greater numbers of physicians into greater numbers of confrontations with malpractice lawyers, state licensing boards, hospitals, health insurers, and patients, and such imbroglios will invariably sap the very strength that physicians need, individually and collectively, to combat the increasing socialization of medicine in America.

This, of course, is unfortunate because medical errors and their political aftermath make strange bedfellows. Physicians need to eliminate medical errors for reasons that transcend those postulated by individuals and groups who stand to profit, materially and/or politically, from the very existence of such mistakes.

Much like the atheist who confused bingo with prayer, many observers are displaying similar confusion over the reasons physicians make errors. Many writers and reporters seem to think that Medicine's many distractions, such as pending malpractice litigation or the multifarious restrictions of managed care, are sufficient to explain why good doctors make bad mistakes.

There is little question that distractions can lead to errors in any profession, but what many observers are overlooking is the major reason why physicians make mistakes, ranging from the miniscule to the tragic. More than distractions or indiscretions, physicians make errors because they have allowed themselves to become too busy.

Due to the very structure of medical education, physicians are forced to be busy throughout the course of their medical school and residency training. As the completion of medical training draws near, residents start to accept being perpetually busy because of the prospect of becoming wealthy and successful as busy physicians.

With personalities frequently altered by the effects of chronic sleep deprivation and values frequently obfuscated by the combined effects of delayed gratification and long-standing indebtedness, many physicians enter the medical workforce with little alternative but to become busy immediately. Unfortunately, after many years of practice, too many physicians continue to work at a hectic, if not frantic, pace.

Financial necessity or the perception thereof, personality traits, fear of losing patients or income, unwillingness or inability to share patients with other health care providers, and simply not knowing any other way to practice medicine are but a few of the many reasons physicians stay busier and work harder than necessary. Unfortunately, it is this exaggerated work ethic that frequently leads to an unhealthy reliance on shortcuts and unsound practice styles.

An alarming number of patients complain about becoming a part of a physician's "assembly line." They resent waiting hours to see a physician who spends only a few minutes with them, who fails to take the time necessary to communicate with them, and who moves swiftly from one examination room to the next—leaving behind a trail of unanswered questions.

The vast majority of patients want a physician who is available to speak to them on the telephone, a physician who takes the time to discuss their progress during hospital rounds, and a physician who doesn't leave patients or their families with the impression that he or she is too busy to discuss matters of health. To many patients, availability is a physician's most important attribute.

Physicians who are too busy to listen to their patients frequently miss information that is important to patient care and risk making serious medical errors that might have been prevented if such information were known. Physicians who are too busy to thoroughly review a patient's chart on a routine basis run the same risk.

Surgeons who remove the wrong lung from a patient or a healthy thyroid from a patient who was hospitalized for a nephrectomy are generally not incompetent physicians. Instead, they are typically physicians who have allowed themselves to become too busy to perform their job safely, and as a result, physicians who have allowed themselves to become prone to serious errors.

By allowing themselves to become too busy, too many physicians create potentially preventable medical errors, deprive their family and friends of their presence and involvement, and frequently neglect or injure their own physical or mental health. In an age when many observers claim that America has a surplus of health care providers, this is both unfortunate and unnecessary.

Instead of mandating the reporting of medical errors, those who purport to be concerned with the safety of health care in America should explore ways to eliminate such errors before they happen. One such way would be to help physicians discover how to reduce their workload, create more time for each patient, and reserve more time for themselves and their families.

As I was finishing my residency in internal medicine, I considered a number of different practice options in a number of different locations. I finally chose a rural setting because I wanted the time to practice medicine at any unfrenzied pace, to pursue a number of different avocations, and most importantly, to spend with my family.

I have never earned the kind of income that physicians practicing in larger cities command, but I have not starved or wanted for much either. Given the option of more money or more time for myself, my family, and my patients, I would always choose more time.

Having extra time has allowed me to maintain my enthusiasm for the practice of medicine. Sufficient time and continued interest in my work have helped me obviate many errors that physicians, who have allowed themselves to become too busy and too distracted, continue to make.

Regardless of programs or mandates, there will always be physicians who practice medicine on an assembly line. These physicians should realize that no one has ever seen a Brink's truck following a hearse in a funeral procession.

Regardless of new options or newer ideas, there will always be physicians who refuse to believe that the medical profession can change for the better. These physicians should realize that there are no atheists in a foxhole.

April, 2000

DYING WITH DIGNITY

His colleagues called him "Doctor Ski." It's not that his Polish surname was that long or difficult to pronounce, but Doctor Ski was a simple man and the name seemed to fit.

A psychiatrist by trade, Doctor Ski was truly one of a kind. He listened long, spoke briefly, and always seemed to understand.

Doctor Ski spoke broken English from behind an elaborate network of shining dental bridges and caps. When he smiled, he gave the appearance of a man who had just been thrown head-first through the antique-metals section of a jewelry store.

If Doctor Ski's dental work was distracting, his style of dress was alarming. His typical work ensemble usually included a checkered coat, plaid slacks, pattern shirt, novelty necktie, and blue vinyl loafers.

There were those who accused Doctor Ski of buying his clothes at thrift shops and yard sales, but the good-natured physician didn't seem to be bothered by such persiflage. As the staff psychiatrist of a rural mental health clinic, Doctor Ski took care of the psychiatric problems of the poor, and like most of his patients, he dressed for comfort rather than fashion.

On his best day, Doctor Ski never resembled a typical psychiatrist, but his practice wasn't a typical psychiatry practice. Doctor Ski took care of the indigent who couldn't afford other psychiatrists, as well as the outcasts who weren't welcome in other psychiatrists' offices, and always in a competent and compassionate manner.

A little over a year ago, Doctor Ski learned that he had metastatic cancer. In an unceremonious fashion, he retired from his practice and dedicated his remaining days to closing out his worldly affairs.

As his disease progressed, Doctor Ski experienced a significant amount of pain, as well as many of the other complications of meta-static disease. Doctor Ski took medication to control his pain and discomfort, but he refused all other medications and life-sustaining treatments.

Doctor Ski remained self-sufficient until his disease reached its final stage. When he became too weak to engage in normal activities and when his medications no longer controlled his pain, he agreed to a terminal hospitalization.

In the week that followed, Doctor Ski accepted parenteral pain medication but nothing else. As he prepared to die, he refused intravenous fluids, food, and anything not directly associated with immediate comfort.

Doctor Ski had always been a simple man. To the final detail, his death was as uncomplicated as his life.

Having been a psychiatrist, Doctor Ski took care of many suicidal patients and counseled many individuals who were contemplating euthanasia. He understood the many ramifications of death and dying, and he could have easily opted for a quick end to his own pain and suffering.

So, why didn't he? It can be argued that Doctor Ski was a religious man—the product of a Judaeo-Christian ethic.

It can also be argued that he was a physician—a man who understood the workings and limitations of the human body and a man who was bound to the prohibitions of the Hippocratic Oath. It can even be argued that he was a peaceful man—a man whose life operated within the framework of established laws and customs.

Perhaps those who knew Doctor Ski best would argue that he was a learned man—a man whose understanding of life's continuum was derived from many different sources and a man who took the time to try to understand the meaning of life and the parameters of destiny. Perhaps those who knew him best would argue that he was an unconventional man—a man not easily influenced by current wisdom or cultural trends.

Because of his peculiar style of dress, Doctor Ski was once described as a "human Rorschach card." Despite such notoriety, he lived and worked with self-assuredness and uncommon dignity.

With a slightly different wardrobe, Doctor Ski could have been a psychiatrist to the rich and famous, but he chose to take care of the poor and disenfranchised. With slightly different priorities, he could have used his profession for personal gain, but he chose to share his holdings and energies with the less fortunate.

Doctor Ski was a simple man who lived his life according to a well-organized set of uncomplicated principles. If his life taught us anything, it was the importance of living with dignity.

Doctor Ski was a consistent man who died the same way he lived. If his death taught us anything, it was the true meaning of dying with dignity.

December, 1994

TEAM PHYSICIANS

It is a little known fact that team physicians, who treat professional or amateur athletes at out-of-state competitions, may be risking criminal and civil liability. Although legal action has never been taken by a state medical board against a visiting team physician, 18 states do not allow team physicians to treat athletes unless they are licensed to practice medicine in the state of the competition, 6 states require out-of-state doctors to apply for a courtesy license before they are allowed to treat athletes, and 16 states allow visiting team physicians to treat athletes only as consultants to home team physicians.

In a recent survey of team physicians from 30 states, 71% of the doctors claimed they were unaware of any state laws that prohibited them from treating athletes at out-of-state competitions, 53% stated they never contacted home team physicians before traveling to out-of-state competitions, and 66% stated they didn't consider themselves to be a consultant to a home team physician. Ergo, many team physicians are still unaware of the potential criminal and civil liability associated with treating athletes away from home.

A number of medical boards that do not allow visiting team physicians to treat athletes within their state borders argue that such physicians are unnecessary and incapable of rendering medical care that cannot be provided by doctors who are already licensed to practice medicine in their state. The medical board members who express this sentiment should have been with me last week-end when I traveled to another state to watch my daughter play in a college softball tournament.

Early in the semi-final game of the tournament, one of my daughter's teammates fell to the ground after being hit in the face with a softball. Because my daughter's team is one of the many Division-One college softball teams that do not travel with a team physician, I was summoned to the field by the team's coach and student trainer.

Although I do not hold a license to practice medicine in the state where the tournament was being held, the player required immediate medical attention and no other physicians were present. Without giving any thought to what codicil of the "Good Samaritan" Law sanctioned my intervention, I rushed to the injured player's side.

When I examined the player, it was apparent that she had sustained a facial laceration and contusion, and was hemorrhaging from both nostrils. She never lost consciousness, her vision and extraocular muscle activity were unimpaired, and her neurological exam, including cranial nerve assessment, was normal.

After I stopped the nasal hemorrhages, treated the superficial laceration, and started to address the problem of facial swelling, I realized the player had probably sustained hairline fractures of facial and nasal bones. Having rendered similar emergency treatment to the same player a year earlier for a nasal fracture that ultimately required surgery, I also realized the importance of team physicians who were not only capable of handling emergencies but also aware of the medical and surgical histories of the individual team members.

If I had not been present at the game, the team's coaching staff would have had little recourse but to have the player evaluated by another physician at a hospital emergency room more than 30 minutes away. Insofar as the team traveled to the tournament by bus, an ambulance would have been required to transport the player to the hospital, and a member of the coaching staff would have been required to accompany the player.

In light of the player's previous fractures and extensive surgery, the interpretation of x-rays or CT scans by an emergency physician or consultant, with or without previous studies for comparison, would have been difficult. With the player being nearly 200 miles from her college campus, she would have been referred back to her personal physician for any non-emergency treatment.

A great deal of time and money would have been spent attempting to evaluate and treat the player's injury in unfamiliar surroundings. In comparison to the immediate informed treatment she received at the time of her injury and emotional support she received from her teammates and coaches, any delayed or unnecessary treatment rendered at an unfamiliar hospital would have been decidedly inferior.

Many professional and amateur athletes with significant medical and surgical histories continue to engage in physically and psychologically demanding athletic competition. This is why team physicians are so important.

Team physicians are capable of handling emergencies when and where they occur, and because of their familiarity with the athletes and their medical histories, they are also capable of providing higher level care. This translates into medical intervention that is more timely, accessible, and cost-effective.

The list of athletes who continue to thrive within the wide world of sports despite asthma, seizure disorders, cardiac arrhythmias, orthopedic injuries, and a whole host of other physical and psychological problems is vast. Were it not for the interest, support, and availability of competent team physicians, many of these athletes would be unable to sustain their athletic careers.

I attended another softball tournament this week-end and got a big hug from a pretty young lady whose hairline facial and nasal fractures have been healing nicely without surgical intervention. She is still disappointed that she wasn't able to help her team win their last few tournaments, but there will be other tournaments, and her surgeon has assured her that she will be playing again in the near future.

The controversy over visiting team physicians treating athletes during out-of-state competitions will probably remain with us for quite some time. What promises to endure longer, however, are the athletic careers and programs that continue to be fortified by team physicians whose many talents include being able to tell one patient from another without a score card.

October, 2000

THE ART OF COMMUNICATING

My wife first met Jimmy when she was only 7 years-old. She remembers him as a kind and considerate man who seemed to enjoy going out of his way to help his neighbors.

She remembers hearing various community leaders praising Jimmy as a war hero and a truly intelligent man. She remembers how he would take all the kids in the neighborhood to the corner store for ice cream and how he would laugh when ice cream covered their faces.

A few years ago, Jimmy retired and moved into the rural community where I practice medicine. On his first visit to my office, his many different medical conditions were readily apparent, but not as apparent as his gentlemanly demeanor.

Jimmy was everything my wife had told me he would be—and more. He was thoughtful, grateful, and the kind of human being whose three-quarters of a century on this mortal coil had made the earth a considerably nicer place.

While traveling a few weeks ago, Jimmy stopped at a diner for breakfast. When he suddenly started to develop slurred speech and motor weakness, an ambulance was called and he was taken to the emergency room of a large hospital.

A CT scan of the brain, which was obtained in the emergency room, demonstrated a brain tumor. After the CT scan and a number of other diagnostic studies had been performed, the ER physician returned to Jimmy's room and unemotionally announced, "We're admitting you to the hospital for treatment of your brain cancer."

Frightened, alone, and unable to move or speak intelligibly, Jimmy had little recourse but to follow the mandates of the physician and undergo hospitalization. A few hours later, as Jimmy was being prepped for bronchoscopy and a bone scan, his family arrived at the hospital.

Upon being informed of the tests that had been scheduled to determine if Jimmy's brain lesion was a primary tumor or a metastasis, the family conferred with Jimmy. After their conference, his family courteously requested that the tests be postponed.

"The consultants are all very upset with you," the admitting internist told Jimmy and his family. "These doctors are very busy and they don't like to have their procedures cancelled."

Although Jimmy's family tried to explain that he was very weak, emotionally upset, and unsure if he wanted to undergo any invasive procedures, the attending physician seemed more concerned about the convenience of his colleagues and the utilization of a hospital bed than the feelings or immediate needs of his patient or his patient's family. The next day, Jimmy was seen by an oncologist.

"From reviewing your tests, it appears that you have a very rapidly growing form of lung cancer that has spread to your brain," the oncologist abruptly informed Jimmy. "This kind of tumor grows so fast that the same x-rays probably wouldn't have picked it up a few months ago."

Instead of giving his elderly patient the opportunity to process some of the information, react, or ask questions, the oncologist just continued his canned speech. "We're going to start radiation therapy, which may not help your cancer and may even make matters worse, but we'll give it a try and see what happens."

For the next few days, Jimmy remained hospitalized and received his scheduled radiation therapy. He saw his physicians daily, but began to dread their insensitive verbal barrages.

Following his long ordeal at the large, impersonal hospital, Jimmy was discharged and sent home. At the present time, he is stable but the effects of his disease are becoming more and more apparent.

In my years of medical training and clinical practice, I have been continually amazed at the incredible number of physicians who lack the ability to effectively communicate with their patients. I have seen physicians whose communications skills lack compassion, understanding, and common courtesy, and whose feeble attempts at communicating with patients have undermined the credibility of the entire medical profession.

It is one thing to be tired, overworked, or even burnt out, but it is quite another thing to be chronically unaware of the responsibilities of one's position in life. Rendering medical care to another human being is a distinct privilege, and awareness of that privilege must be effectively communicated to patients and their families.

Many medical students and residents currently receive formal training in the art of communicating. Unfortunately, such training has not proven to be uniformly successful.

It is one thing for a medical student to have his or her ability to interact with patients critiqued. It is quite another thing for that same student to choose as a role model a medical school professor whose research credits or clinical skills are much more impressive than his or her bedside manner.

Many physicians would think nothing of apprising a colleague of a potentially dangerous medical or surgical practice, but very few physicians would apprise a colleague of poor communications skills. The inability of physicians to effectively communicate with their patients is one of the major reasons for the malpractice epidemic, and as much a threat to the medical profession as clinical incompetence.

There are no good ways to tell a patient that they have cancer, but some ways are better than others. Effective communication is as simple as taking the time to see the person inside the patient and talking to that person in a manner that reflects an understanding of their needs.

Jimmy is a kind old man who did not deserve the arrogant and insensitive medical treatment he recently received. None of our patients do.

October, 1994

MASTERPIECES

A ccording to legend, it took Leonardo da Vinci more than seven years to paint his masterpiece, ***The Last Supper***. During that period of time, he painted the figures of Jesus Christ and each of the twelve apostles individually using real life models.

The artist decided to paint the figure of Christ first. Before he could begin the six-month process, however, da Vinci had to choose a model from hundreds of would-be subjects.

Following lengthy auditions, the master finally chose a nineteen year-old to serve as the model for Christ. He wanted to portray Christ as a man of beauty, strength, and innocence, and only one candidate possessed the unique blend of traits the artist envisioned.

After da Vinci completed the figure of Christ, he held another audition to select the model for the first apostle to be added to his masterpiece. For the next six years, he repeated the process of auditioning models and adding new characters to his painting until all but one figure remained to complete his work of art.

For many weeks, da Vinci searched for a model for the painting's final character, Judas Iscariot. The artist required a subject who appeared contemptible and capable of betraying a close friend, but such a subject was nowhere to be found.

After an exhaustive and disappointing search, da Vinci finally visited a prison in Rome where a convicted murderer was awaiting execution. It took da Vinci only one glance at the mean, troubled, and disheveled criminal to realize that he had finally found his Judas.

By order of the king, the criminal was transported from Rome to Milan. For many months, he remained in Milan where he was incarcerated and taken to da Vinci's studio whenever the artist called.

When da Vinci finally completed his portrayal of Judas Iscariot on canvas, he ordered the guards to return their prisoner to Rome. Hearing the command, the criminal broke away from the guards, grabbed da Vinci, and asked the artist how he could allow an old friend to be returned to prison.

"What do you mean—old friend?" da Vinci inquired. "I have never seen you before that day when I discovered you in prison."

"You have known me longer than that, da Vinci," the criminal cried. "I was the young boy you painted as Christ seven years ago."

Leonardo da Vinci was known as a man of great perception. This should come as no surprise to anyone who has ever studied his art.

Despite his extraordinary perception, however, he failed to detect Christ in the face of Judas. He failed to see the innocent face of a young boy beneath the hardened features of a criminal.

Today, many physicians have developed the habit of only viewing the medical profession at face value. They look at Medicine, but can only see the scars of managed care, the constant threat of malpractice litigation, and the unremitting process of socialization.

Their dilemma is similar to that which perplexed da Vinci in the 15th century. They look at Medicine and see flaws, but not the many hidden qualities that originally attracted them to the profession.

At face value, contemporary American Medicine is a study in imperfections, but beneath its current visage, it is still a masterpiece. There is little question that our profession is currently plagued by many problems and in need of an urgent face lift, but who better to solve the problems and improve Medicine's appearance than those of us who refuse to lose sight of its underlying beauty.

February, 2001

THROWING THE BABY OUT WITH THE BATH WATER

A recent edition of the *American Medical News* ran a cover story, entitled, "AMA Wants Bad Doctors Off Its Membership Rolls." In short, the article chronicled the American Medical Association's recent attempts to expel its members who have been convicted of fraud or felony involving professional misconduct, have had their medical licenses revoked for professional reasons, or have been discharged from the armed forces or government positions because of professional misconduct or incompetence.

When I read the article, I immediately thought of Teddy. Just a few years ago, Teddy was one of the medical profession's fastest rising stars.

He was intelligent, skilled, enthusiastic, personable, and caring. Teddy knew who he was and where he was going, but that was before the incident that turned him into the kind of doctor the AMA wants off its membership rolls.

Following a seemingly uneventful surgical procedure, Teddy reviewed a set of follow-up x-rays and realized that a sponge had been left inside his patient. There was little doubt in Teddy's mind that the foreign body had resulted from the invasive procedure, and there was even less doubt that a disclosure of his findings would result in a malpractice suit.

Teddy knew that retrieval of the foreign body would be difficult, and that his patient was not the sort who handled bad news well. Since the patient was asymptomatic and unaware of the presence of any foreign body, Teddy went against his better judgment and decided to keep quiet about the entire incident.

A number of months later, Teddy realized that he had panicked and that his cover up was a mistake, but his recognition of the obvious was too late. Another physician had already been consulted by the patient, and Teddy's errant ways were quickly uncovered.

What followed could only be described as Medicine's endorsement of the "Domino Theory." Following the disclosure of the entire incident, the patient filed a hefty malpractice suit against Teddy.

The suit led to the loss of Teddy's hospital privileges. In turn, this development led to a state investigation that ultimately led to the suspension of Teddy's medical license.

By the time Teddy's license was finally suspended, he had already started practicing medicine in another state. The news of his suspension spread quickly, and it wasn't long before his new patients were reading shocking stories about their physician in a local newspaper.

On the same night Teddy's wife presented him with a new baby, he was informed that his hospital privileges were being revoked and that his salaried position with the hospital was being terminated. Even though his practice had been exemplary and his unfortunate incident had occurred over three years earlier, the bad publicity forced the hospital to show Teddy the door.

Teddy tried unsuccessfully to open his own practice in the same town, but after his savings were depleted and his wife filed for divorce, he was forced to move on by himself. Teddy managed to land a few emergency room jobs in a number of small hospitals, but his experiences left him with about as much satisfaction as that of a renowned artist who was being paid to paint fences.

Today, Teddy continues to search for his own identity. What's more, he continues to seek forgiveness for the only mistake in his entire professional life, and understanding from his colleagues.

It is ironic that the AMA wants to remove "bad doctors" from its membership rolls when the organization epitomizes the very system that creates bad doctors. For generations, the AMA has watched as medical schools have bestowed neuroses and physical afflictions on would-be doctors by using intimidating and poorly-focused educational methods.

The AMA has also watched as internship and residency training programs have altered the personalities of young physicians by feeding them a strict diet of sleep deprivation and unrealistic professional expectations. By repeatedly kowtowing to the federal government and by not fighting for the civil rights of its members, the AMA has exposed physicians to a stressful professional milieu in which heroism is rewarded with malpractice suits, respect for human dignity is rewarded with the red tape of Medicare and the red ink of Medicaid, and dedication is rewarded with the wrath of the American public.

Medicine is, arguably, this nation's most demanding profession. If it weren't, an inordinately high percentage of physicians wouldn't continue to be the victims of suicide and other forms of premature death, an unacceptably high percentage of physicians wouldn't continue to succumb to the effects of alcoholism and drug addiction, and a regrettably high percentage of physicians wouldn't continue to rely on divorce as a means of explaining the incongruity between their professional and personal lives.

Contrary to the AMA's opinion, there are no bad doctors. There are only good doctors who are forced into bad situations by their own human nature and by the imperfections of the system that employs them.

"A doctor is a man, Ben Casey," Doctor Zorba was fond of reminding his student. Accordingly, mistakes are as much the birth right of any doctor as they are of any other man.

No one can ever condone the kind of mistake Teddy made. What everyone can do, however, is understand that some mistakes are worse than others, but a mistake is a mistake, and no human being is immune from making them.

As Teddy's story will readily attest, the medical profession has gotten very good at "throwing the baby out with the bath water." In its haste to comply with society's misdirection, the medical profession has turned its backs on members who would venture from the straight and narrow.

If all of us in Medicine are to successfully handle the profound external problems that are currently confronting our profession, we must first develop a renewed sense of internal strength. We must find ways for physicians like Teddy to handle their problems without having to forfeit their membership in the medical profession, and we must also find ways to prevent other physicians from developing similar problems.

We must learn how to embrace the axiomatic, "Physician, Heal Thyself," and expand it into the more timely, "Physicians, Heal Thyselves." If all of us in Medicine expect to see our profession regain the prestige it once had, we must stop turning impaired physicians into pariahs and start redirecting our energies against the outside forces in society that would have us do so.

To this end, we must stop confusing malpractice with maloccurrence, and finally acknowledge that one can be corrected through education while the other must be redefined through legislation. We must stop listening to those who would have the medical profession abandon its members, who have contracted such diseases as AIDS, and reassert our right to develop health care policy rather than follow it.

If any of us in Medicine are ever to realize the dream which brought us into the profession, we must start rethinking many of our established practices. We must rethink censuring, sanctioning, and suspending, just as we must rethink hospital privileges, peer review, and expert testimony.

A chain is only as strong as its weakest link. Accordingly, the medical profession can only regain its former strength if every physician is willing to share his or her strength with those colleagues who have temporarily lost their own.

The AMA may go ahead with its plans and remove those doctors it considers "bad" from its membership rolls, but the medical profession will be no better for the decision. Each time it thoughtlessly expels one of its members, the AMA risks throwing the baby out with the bath water.

December, 1991

THE BOSTON TEA
PARTIES

I n 1767, the British government enacted the Townshend Acts to assert imperial authority in America by means of taxation and customs enforcement. In 1770, following many violent protests by American colonists, the Brits repealed the duties on such commodities as paint, glass, and paper, but continued to levy an import tax on tea.

In 1773, the British Parliament enacted the Tea Act which granted marketing privileges to the British East India Company and allowed a small group of merchants to monopolize on American tea trade. A group of American colonists protested the Tea Act by staging the Boston Tea Party.

On the evening of December 16, 1773, colonists disguised as Indians boarded three ships in Boston Harbor and dumped 342 chests of tea overboard. The Boston Tea Party officially protested Britain's Tea Act and set the stage for similar tea parties in other American cities.

In 1774, in direct response to the Boston Tea Party, the British Parliament enacted the so-called Intolerable or Coercive Acts. Among other restrictions, the Intolerable Acts closed Boston Harbor to commercial traffic pending reimbursement for the destroyed tea, greatly increased the law enforcement and judicial powers of British officials in America, banned unauthorized town meetings by colonists, permitted a change of venue for British officials charged with criminal offenses in America, and authorized the quartering of British troops in American houses and buildings.

Collectively, the Intolerable Acts served as the final straw that broke the camel's back. American outrage over the Intolerable Acts led to the

First Continental Congress which, in turn, led to American independence from England and the birth of the United States of America.

In the final decades of the twentieth century, the federal government of the United States enacted various laws to assert its authority over health care in America. Realizing that tremendous profits were to be had from an emerging one-trillion dollar health care industry, representatives of the federal government had earlier conspired with powerful businessmen to create managed care—a form of socialized medicine that sanctioned corporate profiteering through a system of health care rationing to patients and fee rationing to physicians.

A few of the laws that were written to help politicians, businessmen, and investors reap the profits from American health care were the Employee Retirement Income Security Act (ERISA) which protected managed care from malpractice litigation, the McCarran-Ferguson Act which exempted managed care from antitrust laws, and the Health Maintenance Organization Act which protected managed care from unfavorable taxation. In addition to these laws, many other governmental regulations were promulgated to facilitate the workings of managed care.

Following many individual and collective protests by American physicians and health care consumers, the federal government formed various committees and compiled various guidelines to create the illusion that managed care was being closely watched and regulated. With the apparent realization that the government's committees were little more than lip service and their guidelines little more than window dressing, a group of physicians and nurses calling themselves the "Ad Hoc Committee To Defend Health Care" gathered on Griffin's Wharf in Boston on December 2, 1997 for a reenactment of the Boston Tea Party.

From the deck of the good ship, ***Beaver***, these latter-day "Sons and Daughters of Liberty" tossed symbolic crates into Boston Harbor. Although the crates were later retrieved, their temporary presence atop Boston's waters conveyed a message no less meaningful or urgent than that conveyed by tea crates two centuries earlier.

As they tossed their symbolic crates overboard, the members of the Ad Hoc Committee To Defend Health Care shouted that Medicine should not be diverted from its primary tasks of relieving suffering, preventing and treating illness, and promoting health. They also clamored that there was no room in caregiving for corporate profit or personal fortune.

As they continued to jettison the ship's cargo, the committee members protested that financial incentives rewarding overcare or undercare must be prohibited, that the right of patients to choose their own physicians must be insured, and that universal coverage must be guaranteed as a matter of national policy. By the time the last crate had been dumped into the frigid water, the doctors and nurses of the Ad Hoc Committee had told the world exactly what was wrong with managed care.

Inevitably, the reenactment of the Boston Tea Party will set the stage for similar tea parties and similar protests by other groups of physicians in other American cities. Predictably, such events will also set the stage for retaliation by the federal government and the insurance industry.

As health care profiteering by government and big business becomes more and more threatened by the protests of physicians and patients, it is inevitable that government will enact a modern-day version of the Intolerable Acts to keep the medical profession at bay. As this occurs, it is also inevitable that a greater number of physicians will join the fight against managed care and the socialization of medicine in America.

If history can be expected to repeat itself, an army of discontent physicians will one day create a congress of sorts or a union that is dedicated to preserving the practice of medicine and returning American medicine to its rightful owners. This, in effect, will wrest medicine from the politicians, businessmen, and profiteers, and quickly restore America's traditional doctor-patient relationship.

Townshend Acts, Tea Acts, and Intolerable Acts were not tolerated by our forefathers, and with time, managed care will no longer be tolerated by the American medical profession or the millions we serve. With each new passing day, more and more physicians are starting to come to the realization that managed care just isn't our cup of tea!

January, 1998

PHYSICIAN-ASSISTED SUICIDE

I first met Kay a little over a year ago when she came to my office complaining of vague hypogastric pressure. When I referred the obese, fifty year-old woman to a gynecologist, a large fibroid tumor was discovered and an elective hysterectomy was scheduled at a major medical center.

Kay reported to the hospital expecting a relatively simple surgical procedure and a short hospital stay. Her surgical procedure was begun but quickly aborted when metastatic ovarian carcinoma was discovered.

Kay's post-operative course was a nightmare. She had a near-fatal reaction to chemotherapy, followed by the development of deep vein thrombophlebitis in her left calf, uncontrollable diabetes, fever of unknown origin, and two separate entero-cutaneous fistulas that drained from her abdominal wall.

When it became increasingly difficult for Kay to find a physician to talk to or a nurse to inject her overdue pain medications, Kay began to wonder if she would not be better off dead. Somehow, Kay survived the hospitalization and returned home after she was told that nothing else could be done for her at the renowned medical center.

Kay returned home with the belief that her husband and son continued to bring meaning and purpose to her life, and with the understanding that each additional day of life was a bonus. For the past eight months, I have been trying to support her belief by making weekly visits to Kay's home.

Although her disease has progressed, Kay's pain has been well controlled, and she has been able to function surprisingly well within the confines of her home. For Kay, simple things like feeling the warmth of the sun on her face or smelling a freshly-picked rose have taken on new importance and have reminded her of what a precious gift life really is.

When I visited Kay this morning, she was watching a news report on Jack Kevorkian's latest attempts at physician-assisted suicide. As I watched the report with Kay and her husband, I felt as though I had just stepped into a magnetic field.

At one pole, a well known advocate of suicide was talking about helping people prematurely end their own lives. At the other pole, a patient was discussing her terminal illness and the therapy that would hopefully allow her to see the light of yet another day.

One of the medical profession's most pressing issues is whether or not physicians should help patients commit suicide. The issue here is not one of physicians opting not to provide life-sustaining treatment to terminally-ill patients, but rather one of assisting patients in the termination of their own lives.

The former is a humane and medically-ethical gesture. The latter is a thoroughly illegal and immoral activity.

Because the vast majority of American physicians have had their moral values shaped by a Judeo-Christian ethic, it would appear that the religious heritage of the American medical profession would cast a loud vote against physician-assisted suicide. The admonition, "Thou Shalt Not Kill," clearly prohibits the taking of human life.

Because the vast majority of American physicians have taken the Hippocratic Oath, it would also appear that the time-honored ethical tradition of the medical profession would cast yet another vote against physician-assisted suicide. As the Hippocratic Oath proclaims, "I will give no deadly medicine to any one if asked, nor suggest any such counsel......"

Law, religion, and tradition notwithstanding, it would appear that physician-assisted suicide is inconsistent with the fundamental purpose of the medical profession. As physicians, we must all be champions of life and reserve the termination of life to that power from which all life emanates.

If life was perfect, there would be no pain or suffering. If life was perfect, there would be no need for compassionate human beings to devote their entire lives to mastering an imperfect science that inconsistently succeeds at relieving mankind's pain and suffering.

Unfortunately, life is not perfect. Herein lies our individual and collective purposes as physicians.

In a society of diverse roles and arcane practices, there may be a need for someone to assist others in the termination of life. As long as Kay and others like her express a willingness to glean yet another precious moment from their lives, however, I will not believe that the "someone" has to be a physician.

December, 1992

HARD WORK AND SACRIFICE

A skilled but discontented gynecologist secretly took a night course to become an auto mechanic. Following the course and a lengthy practical exam, he eagerly awaited his test score in the mail.

The gynecologist was surprised when he received a final grade of 150. Somewhat confused, he called his instructor.

The instructor explained to the gynecologist that he received 50 points for successfully removing the engine from the test vehicle and another 50 points for successfully replacing the engine. When the instructor was asked about the 50 bonus points, he told the gynecologist that the points were awarded for degree of difficulty.

"I felt it was only fair to give you the extra points," the instructor told the gynecologist. "You were the only student in the class who removed and replaced the engine through the tail pipe!"

My oldest son just completed his first year of medical school. He is spending the summer seeing patients with me in my office.

My daughter just finished her third year as a pre-med student in college. She is spending the summer compiling patients' records in my office and using the opportunity to learn medicine's vocabulary.

When my oldest son is not helping me see patients, he is helping my daughter prepare for the Medical College Admissions Test she will be taking at the end of the summer. She was unable to take the exam this past spring because she plays college softball to help finance her college education.

My youngest son starts college this fall. Like my oldest son and daughter, he will also study pre-med, play a sport at the Division-One level, and help finance his own education through scholarships.

It seems that my three children are always studying, playing a sport, or helping each other achieve their mutual goals. They are all very successful, but they work very hard to achieve their success.

I don't know a single physician who didn't work hard or make untold sacrifices to become a doctor. The hard work and sacrifice started in college, intensified in medical school, and escalated during residency training.

What's more, I don't know a single physician who didn't continue to work hard and make sacrifices throughout his or her medical career. It is one thing to reach the top of the mountain, but quite another thing to be able to cling to the peak for more than an instant.

Too many physicians have forgotten how hard they worked and how much they sacrificed to become a doctor. They have also forgotten how indispensable physicians are to society and the power doctors possess.

Government, the insurance industry, and legal profession have joined forces to keep physicians under society's thumb. They have tried to convince physicians that a car's engine can only be viewed through the tail pipe.

The time has come for every physician to recall the hard work and sacrifices that allowed us to join the world's most coveted profession. The time has come for physicians to stop settling for sneak peaks through the tail pipe of a car we already own.

August, 2001

TOO MANY PHYSICIANS

This morning, as I was trying to clear my desk of some leftover paperwork, a few unexpected visitors came to my office. The minister and his wife had just recently moved to upstate New York, and as I looked at their smiling faces through the frosted window of my office door, I began to wonder why they had chosen a snowy Saturday morning for a return trip to the mountains of Northeastern Pennsylvania.

Following the customary round of "hi's," and "howdy do's," the minister's wife began to talk about a current illness that was causing her and her husband no undo trepidation. Between paroxysms of coughing, she talked about a two-month upper respiratory tract infection that just did not seem to be getting any better.

When she first realized that she had an infection that required medical attention, she called a nearby medical clinic, but was told that she would have to wait a few days for the earliest appointment. When she finally visited the medical clinic, she was seen by a physician's assistant.

Following a progressively downhill course that was marked by a number of unsuccessful therapeutic interventions and the eventual discovery that her caregiver was not a physician, she demanded to be seen by a medical doctor. Despite the physician's assurance that the next round of antibiotics, inhalers, and decongestants would do the trick, her condition continued to worsen.

As I examined her, she joked that, when she finally regained her strength, she planned to be angry at the recent course of events in her life. Considering her prolonged wait to be seen for an acute illness, her not being immediately informed that she would be seen by a physician's assistant rather than a medical doctor, her being charged the same amount of money to see a physician's assistant as she was charged to see a medical doctor, a staggering pharmacy bill, a seven-day absence from work, and an inadequately diagnosed and incompletely treated illness of two months duration, she has every right to be angry.

When asked if she thought that there were too many doctors in America, she looked at me in disbelief. Her reply was, "Are you joking?"

As a part of his ministry, her husband has made it a practice to accompany members of his church to emergency rooms during periods of critical illness. Prior to recent months, he made it a practice to wait in the emergency room with the patient and the patient's family until treatment was rendered.

The minister still accompanies patients to emergency rooms. Unfortunately, he is no longer able to wait until the patient is seen by a physician.

"In the past year, I've taken many different patients to three different emergency rooms and waited an average of six hours for the patients to be seen by a physician," he said. "I'm happy to take patients to the hospital but I just can't spend a whole day in an emergency room waiting for these people to be seen."

When asked if he thought that there were too many doctors in America, the minister just laughed. His reply was, "You've got to be kidding!"

A few weeks ago, *CNN* ran a story that suggested that there were too many doctors, nurses, and pharmacists in America. The report featured one study recommending that our numbers be reduced by 10% over the next 5 years.

A few months ago, the ***Medical Tribune*** published an article that also suggested a physician oversupply in America. The article recommended limiting the number of foreign medical graduates who train in American hospitals as a method of curbing our purported physician excess.

With another presidential election year upon us, the future of health care in America promises to be the political issue of the day. Health care reform has become the political football in America, and 1996 will undoubtedly find politicians, propagandists, and assorted persona from the special interest sector passing, fumbling, and kicking the political pigskin until it has finally lost its air, laces, and all other defining characteristics.

Before anyone decides that there are too many physicians in America, they would do well to consider a few incontrovertible facts. For starters, Americans are living longer, and the longer they live, the more medical care they will require.

Barring a major catastrophe, natural or unnatural, the earliest years of the 21st Century should find the United States calling itself home to twice as many senior citizens as teenagers. To complicate matters, the number of Americans afflicted with Alzheimer's disease is expected to quadruple within the next fifty years.

Unless a cure for this disease is found, more elderly Americans are expected to contract this dementing illness and require a greater amount of medical care. Likewise, a greater number of Americans will be forced to care for spouses who have contracted Alzheimer's disease, and the stress of taking care of debilitated spouses will also increase the number of illnesses and health care requirements of their caregivers.

With no cure in sight, AIDS, a disease which has already been diagnosed in over one-half million Americans, is expected to complicate matters even more. AIDS affects young and old Americans alike, and as the number of Americans with AIDS continues to increase, greater amounts of medical care will be required.

Simply put, there are not too many physicians in America. What's more, America will continue to need progressively greater numbers of physicians.

Insofar as a greater number of elderly and disabled Americans will require health care in the future, our legislators should rethink their plan to cut hundreds of millions of dollars from the Medicare program. This is especially important in light of the concomitant cuts in the veteran's health programs which could conceivably force hundreds of thousands of American veterans to turn to the Medicare program for their health care.

Careful thought should also be given to cutting funding to the Medicaid program. It is projected that there will be 45-million Americans eligible for the Medicaid program by the year 2005, and less will simply not provide health care for more.

While calm and deliberate consideration is being given to other items on the health care agenda, the same consideration should be given to America's physicians and physician extenders. For the former, it should be realized that physicians cannot be expected to take repeated pay cuts while the cost of living continues to escalate; for the latter, it should be remembered that the role of the physician extender is to assist and not to replace the physician.

Nurse practitioners and physicians assistants cannot be expected, with one-third the formal training of a physician, to function in the same capacity as a physician. Expecting physician extenders to do so is unfair to patients, unfair to physicians, and most assuredly, unfair to the well-meaning nurse practitioners and physicians assistants who, in too many instances, are being forced to work outside the boundaries of their training and competence.

Given the choice between too many and too few physicians in America, I would, without hesitation, choose too many. If there were too many physicians in America, the laws of supply and demand would dominate, allowing only the fittest physicians to survive in the health care marketplace.

On the other hand, if there were too few physicians in America, health care would have to be rationed. Acutely ill patients would have to wait for days to be seen in a clinic by a physician extender and weeks to be seen in the same facility by a physician, and critically ill patients would have to wait for hours to receive life-saving treatment in a hospital emergency room.

Don't look now but health care is already being rationed in the United States. With all due respect to the politicians, propagandists and profiteers, this could only mean that there are not too many physicians in America.

There could never be too many.

December, 1995

LIFE

"**S**ave the whales,...save the whales," Cheech and Chong sing in their movie, ***Nice Dreams***. "Save the whales—but shoot the seals!"

Although the lyrics of Cheech and Chong are not often quoted in the medical literature, their sentiments toward our aquatic friends raise an important issue. Simply put, the ethical values of our society are frequently inconsistent and illogical, as evidenced by our views on life.

For example, there are many people who attempt to protect animals by posting "Save The Whales" bumper stickers on their expensive cars, joining protest marches against the manufacturers and retailers of fur coats, and even refusing to eat meat. Interestingly, many of these same people also support the right to abortion on demand.

There are also many people who actively oppose abortion. Curiously, many in the anti-abortion camp associate with individuals who would protect the life of the unborn at the expense of the lives and well-being of those who participate in the abortion process.

There are others who oppose abortion but support physician-assisted suicide and the death penalty. There are still others who view physician-assisted suicide as murder but the death penalty as the just act of a righteous society.

Additionally, there are those who are against the death penalty but who view physician-assisted suicide as a humane gesture. The comparisons go on and on.

What all this reveals is that, as a society, we tend to be eclectic in our morality. Unfortunately, this picking and choosing of moral values has left us with a cultural neurosis that frequently interferes with our collective ability to clearly identify our beliefs.

As Americans, we have been endowed with the freedom to believe whatever we want. Unfortunately, this same freedom has permitted an abrogation of our responsibility to think critically, logically, and with intellectual consistency.

If logic and consistency are the measure, how can an individual, claiming to be "pro-life," defend the life of the unborn, and at the same time, fail to defend the life of the elderly, the infirm, or the condemned? How can any individual believe that the life of one human being, born or unborn, has any more meaning than the life of any other?

As physicians, we are right in the middle of the ethical controversies and moral dilemmas of our age. Unfortunately, as a profession, we are just as divided on these issues as the society we serve.

Once upon a time, the Hippocratic Oath guided physicians through their moral quandaries. Today, most physicians pick and choose from the Oath, professing that which is least offensive and disregarding the rest.

The medical profession's lack of uniform acceptance of the Hippocratic Oath and its failure to replace the Oath with an alternate standard has helped fuel the cultural neurosis of our society. Physicians have traditionally been expected by society to be champions of life, but in a society that is preparing to embark on a new century with unprecedented freedom and uncertain beliefs, the role of the physician in a new and different world has yet to be defined.

Today, as physicians, we hear laymen defending abortion as though pregnancy following rape was a statistical reality and as though our profession still had not developed ways to effectively handle high risk pregnancies. We hear laymen advocating physician-assisted suicide as though our profession did not know how to control pain and as though we still had not developed effective and compassionate ways to treat the terminally ill.

We hear laymen talking about capital punishment and lethal injection as though physicians should become society's executioners. We hear laymen taking as though suitable alternatives to the death penalty were not available.

Perhaps the time has come for more physicians to start speaking out on matters medical and for more laymen to start listening. Perhaps the time has come for the medical profession to start guiding society instead of allowing itself to be led down society's inconsistent and illogical path.

In my own idealistic world, I see the physician as a champion of life. I also see the physician as someone who is willing to protect life from its initial stages to its natural terminus.

I see the physician as someone who is pro-life. I also see the term, pro-life, being expanded to mean a respect for all human existence.

I am well aware of the fact that there are those who do not share my idealistic view of life. I am also aware of the fact that we live in a crazy world where certain people march in protest of the fur industry, wearing shoes made of alligator leather.

Human life is a precious gift that is ours to cherish and protect, but not to prematurely terminate. So, while we are all busy saving the whales, maybe we should give a little more thought to saving a few more members of our own genus and species—and, of course, the seals!

March, 1995

A HANDFUL OF PILLS

I helped Annie get through her first heart attack 12 years ago. Since that time, I have helped her get through a number of other myocardial infarctions, as well as two cerebrovascular accidents and the death of her husband.

I have also helped her with her Parkinson's disease, diabetes mellitus, hypertension, congestive heart failure, cor pulmonale, emphysema, osteoarthritis, diverticular disease, hepatic dysfunction, peptic ulcer disease, lumbo-sacral disc herniations, uterine carcinoma, and depression. In the past 12 years, Annie and I have been through a lot together.

Annie turned 72 a few weeks ago, and as a birthday present, she received official notification that her participation in a state pharmaceutical assistance program for the elderly was being terminated because her financial assets exceeded program limits by a few hundred dollars. After she read the notification, she began to worry about her inability to afford her numerous medications.

Before she even had the chance to open the rest of her birthday mail, she began to develop severe chest pain. One myocardial infarction later, she found herself celebrating the anniversary of her birth in a hospital intensive care unit.

With the exception of some mental confusion, Annie's hospital stay was unremarkable. Unfortunately, when she returned home, without any further confusion to protect her, she was forced to deal with the reality that her pharmaceutical assistance card was being taken away.

This realization led to a prompt recurrence of her angina. It also led to a prompt deterioration in her overall health.

Annie has been a widow for the past 7 years, but she has been fortunate to have a number of concerned brothers and sisters who have been willing to assist with her health care. One of her sisters called today to tell me that Annie started experiencing severe chest pain while she was talking to her family about the loss of her drug card.

Sensing urgency in her sister's voice, I immediately drove to Annie's home. Annie has never impressed me as being a person of excessive means, and as I stepped inside her home for the first time, I realized that she was living at a bare subsistence level.

Annie's home was old and drafty. Other than a scattering of family photographs, her walls were unadorned.

Stepping inside her living room, I saw Annie lying on an old couch and her brother and two sisters sitting nearby in a variety of poorly matching chairs. Annie complained of chest pressure, as well as slight difficulty breathing and nausea.

After I examined Annie, I expressed my concerns about an extension of her recent myocardial infarction and offered to readmit her to the hospital. Annie tried hard to smile, and grabbing my hand, she graciously declined my offer.

When I asked her why, she told me that she would be more comfortable at home, and then she mumbled something about Medicare not wanting to pay for any more of her hospitalizations. I told Annie that Medicare had no choice but to pay for the hospitalization of a patient with a potentially life-threatening illness, but Annie was not interested in being admitted to any hospital for any reason.

As we talked, her brother and sisters informed me that they had discussed hospitalization with Annie before I arrived and that Annie had expressed the same unwillingness to be hospitalized. They also informed me that they had already arranged for someone to stay with Annie around the clock and that they would call me if her condition changed.

Agreeing to care for Annie at home, I recommended that oxygen be brought in to facilitate her breathing. In the middle of my recommendation, Annie argued that she did not have the money to pay for oxygen.

When I told her that Medicare would pay for it, she protested that Medicare refused to pay for oxygen for her emphysematous sister because of arterial blood gases that did not meet Medicare's rigorous criteria. When I explained the reasons Medicare would pay for the use of oxygen by a patient with multiple life-threatening illnesses, Annie finally permitted me to call for an oxygen concentrator.

When I recommended the use of prochlorperazine suppositories to help combat her severe nausea and nitroglycerin patches to help control her chest pain until she was able to take nitroglycerin capsules by mouth, she once again argued that she would have to do without both medications because she could not afford them. I was finally able to get in a last word with Annie when I remembered that I had samples of both medications in my office and offered to give them to her.

When I left Annie this afternoon, I did so with the realization that I might never see her again, or joke with her again, or have to con her into obtaining badly-needed medical care again. I also left her with the realization that, once upon a time, someone promised Annie that her health care needs would be taken care of when she was no longer able to take care of them herself.

Annie, and millions like her, were there when our nation was still experiencing growing pains. They held America's hand as it struggled through wars, depressions, and disasters.

A handful of pills seem like a small price to pay in return.

October, 1992

CRUISES

The year was 1980, and the place was the lido deck of a cruise ship headed for Bermuda. As I worked hard at getting a sun tan and even harder at trying to forget the residency program I had to return to in one short week, a rotund passenger wiggled his way through a deck of occupied lounge chairs, positioned himself between me and the sun, and loudly proclaimed: "Why, You're Doctor Remakus!"

Just then, the sea gulls quietly came to rest on the deck rails, the steel drum band stopped playing *Jamaica Farewell,* and a few hundred sun-worshipers stared at me as though I was the renowned physician who had invented the vaginal delivery. A few near-sighted men nodded their approval from the other side of the deck, a few semi-attractive ladies smiled from behind the miniature parasols in their tropical drinks, and the corpulent passenger who started all the fuss momentarily sent my wife air-borne by plopping down on the end of her lounge chair.

As the Captain ordered the ship's engines restarted, as calypso music once again filled the air, and as the passengers returned to their previous activities, my uninvited guest proceeded to explain that he had been a patient at the hospital where I was a resident and remembered seeing me working in the hospital's intensive care unit. He also proceeded to tell me all about his pacemaker and how his private physician insisted that he have the pacemaker checked while on he was on his cruise.

I still remember how he placed two fingers on his radial pulse and impersonated the ship's Dutch physician purportedly performing a pacemaker check. "Ya, ya, eees goot," the would-be impersonator bellowed in a blustery tone of voice.

Over the past dozen years, I have taken a number of different cruises and developed an interest in how medicine is practiced at sea. I have been at sea during three different hurricanes, seen many different medical and surgical emergencies aboard ship, and been amazed at the incredible number of misconceptions that both physicians and patients have about cruising.

So, if you are considering going on a cruise yourself, or giving medical advice to patients who are thinking about taking a cruise, here are a few points worth considering. These tips may be of particular help to those who are about to take to the high seas for the first time.

First of all, cruises are among the most popular, most relaxing, and most economical vacations available, and just as well suited for family vacations as they are for quiet getaways. Today, you can cruise just about anywhere in the world and experience the jungles of the Amazon, the glaciers of Alaska, or the islands of the Caribbean.

However, unless you have been endowed with uncommon patience, your cruise experience will only be as good as your choice of ships. There are numerous cruise ships currently at sea, but no two are identical or capable of satisfying every passenger's needs and expectations in the same manner.

After you have picked your destination and talked to your travel agent about the various ships that call on the ports you have chosen, your next call should be to the Centers For Disease Control in Atlanta. Your travel agent may be able to tell you which ship is cheaper or which ship has a polka band, but only the CDC can provide you with timely information concerning the sanitation records and abnormal gastroenteritis rates of all ships which either leave from or arrive at U.S. ports.

As far as the cruise industry is concerned, not all ships are created equal, and certain ships are frequently cited for poor sanitation and above-average rates of gastroenteritis. There is nothing worse than experiencing gastroenteritis at sea, especially when such an unpleasant experience can be potentially avoided by selecting a cruise ship with a clean bill of health.

It is ironic that the ships of one cruise line that currently books a large percentage of medical conventions have also been regulars on the CDC's list of ships with unacceptably high gastroenteritis rates! Maybe there is some truth to the belief that physicians are endowed with a special kind of intestinal fortitude!

After you have selected your ship, an important consideration is the time when you take your cruise. Cruises are usually priced according to seasons with fair-weather or "peak" seasons commanding the highest prices and hurricane or "value" seasons priced significantly lower.

Cruises lines cannot guarantee weather, but rough seas are more likely to be experienced during the hurricane or value season. This may not be a major consideration to a healthy, experienced sea-farer, but it certainly should be to anyone with significant health problems.

Hurricanes at sea are much more fun in retrospect. More than one physician has wished that he had stayed home and studied the new Medicare billing codes instead of deciding to rock and roll with an angry sea.

Another important consideration is your choice of cabin. Cruise prices vary widely according to the size and location of the cabin you select.

Although cabin choice may not be terribly important to an old salt who knows his way around a ship, it can be critically important to passengers with special health requirements. For example, passengers with chronic, debilitating illnesses should select cabins that are located on the main decks, close to the dining rooms and areas of major activity.

Passengers who require wheel chairs or walkers should select cabins as close to elevators as possible. Passengers who suffer from claustrophobia should select outside cabins with port holes, while passengers who suffer from motion sickness should choose inside cabins where motion is less noticeable.

Although every cruise ship has its own physician and infirmary, the abilities of the various physicians and the capabilities of the various infirmaries vary greatly. Most cruise ships can handle minor emergencies and garden variety medical problems, but complicated medical or surgical problems are generally beyond their capability.

Patients with serious medical or surgical problems are generally stabilized until the ship docks and the patient can be transferred to a hospital. In certain rare situations, however, a critically ill patient may be airlifted from the ship.

Among the most common medical problems I have seen at sea are fluid retention caused by drinking desalinated ocean water, gastrointestinal problems caused by dietary indiscretion or infectious gastroenteritis, serious sunburns, incapacitating motion sickness, and orthopedic injuries in passengers who tried to navigate decks and stairwells during rough seas. Some of these problems were unavoidable, but many others could have been prevented with a small dose of foresight.

Simply knowing, for example, that the better cruise ships are willing to use more fuel to keep their stabilizers operative for longer periods of time is valuable information for someone who is prone to motion sickness. It has been said that "you get what you pay for," and nowhere is this more apparent than in the cruise industry.

As you read this article, I'm on a cruise ship that is currently docked at King's Wharf in Bermuda. So, if you are too and you happen to notice a wild and crazy guy doing the limbo with a beautiful girl on each arm and a drink clenched in his teeth—it's not me.

You can find me up on the lido deck. I'm the guy who is squeezing lemon into his iced tea and trying to figure out the new Medicare billing codes!

July, 1992

TALKING ABOUT OUR MISTAKES

A short time ago, one of my elderly patients underwent, what she thought would be, routine cataract surgery. Unfortunately, the outcome of the surgery was anything but routine.

In the days that followed the operation, she noticed that her vision was not improving but progressively deteriorating instead. After a few visits to her ophthalmologist, she finally learned that the wrong intraocular lens had been implanted during surgery.

Not having been present at any of the meetings between the patient and her ophthalmologist, I do not know exactly what was said. I do know, however, that the patient and her husband left the meetings with the distinct impression that the ophthalmologist was trying to convince them that having the wrong intraocular lens implanted during cataract surgery was a relatively common occurrence.

The patient and her husband had planned to spend the winter in Arizona following the surgery, and the ophthalmologist told them that there was no reason for them to change their plans. However, appropriate follow-up with an ophthalmologist in that state was not arranged.

Instead, the patient was casually told that she could have her lens replaced by the ophthalmologist of her choice when she arrived in Arizona. The patient was surprised to hear the ophthalmologist talk about corrective surgery as though it would be as easy as picking out a new pair of reading glasses.

A few months later, the patient underwent a second surgery to have the correct intraocular lens implanted. A few weeks after surgery, she sustained a massive myocardial infarction, which she attributed to the stress of vision loss and multiple surgical procedures.

Somehow, the patient survived the ordeal, and upon returning home, she called me to discuss the entire matter. She was angry at the recent course of events in her life, placing the entire blame for her misfortune on the ophthalmologist who implanted the wrong lens, and demanding satisfaction.

When the patient and her husband started talking about suing the ophthalmologist for malpractice, I gave them some advice from my book, *The Malpractice Epidemic*: "If you or your family ever receive medical treatment which results in a less-than-optimal outcome, make the doctor's office the first place you visit to voice your concern."

For many reasons, this advice made sense to the couple. They were financially-secure individuals who weren't looking forward to making some lawyer rich at the expense of a physician; they just wanted to hear the ophthalmologist admit that he had made a mistake and that he was sorry for the many consequences of that mistake.

I did not know the ophthalmologist, but I naturally assumed that any physician would welcome the opportunity to resolve a potential malpractice suit in his own office instead of a courtroom. Consequently, I was greatly surprised when I learned that the ophthalmologist refused to meet with the patient and her husband.

Undaunted by the refusal of the ophthalmologist to meet with them, the couple decided to visit his office without an appointment. The unannounced visit caught the ophthalmologist off guard, and in the process, answered many of the couple's questions.

According to the patient, the ophthalmologist was defensive and quick to blame the hospital, the lens manufacturer, and even a computer programmer for the surgical blunder. Unfortunately, he was not as quick to offer any apologies or solutions to the problem at hand.

With little alternative, the patient and her husband contacted a lawyer and a malpractice suit was filed against the ophthalmologist. A few months later, the parties settled out of court for a sizeable amount.

Following their settlement, I asked the patient what it would have taken for not to have sued the ophthalmologist. "Hearing him say that he had made a mistake and that he was sorry," she answered without hesitation.

Newsweek recently featured an article written by a teacher whose father died from unexpected complications of elective orthopedic surgery. In this article, the teacher talked about forestalling the distant thunder of litigation, and deciding to meet with his father's surgeons to discover the circumstances surrounding his father's death.

The teacher described his father's two orthopedic surgeons, not as gods or magicians, but as imperfect and fallible men who were frightened to appear so in a society that expected perfection and infallibility from its doctors. Following their meeting, the teacher felt that the surgeons hadn't been negligent or incompetent, but had merely used the complex and dangerous tools of their craft as carefully as they could.

The teacher realized that he could become a millionaire by suing his father's hospital and surgeons. He decided not to file a malpractice suit, however, because he felt it was wrong to sue someone for failing to be the god society expected them to be.

Most lawyers and insurance companies advise physicians never to discuss potential litigation with their patients, and never to admit to a patient that they made a mistake. Similarly, most lawyers advise patients, who have been injured medically or surgically, never to discuss the matter with their physician.

The reason is obvious. If potential plaintiffs and defendants start resolving their differences themselves, a whole bunch of lawyers will have a difficult time maintaining the lifestyle to which they have become accustomed.

And yet, in an earlier day and age when physicians and patients seemed to be reading from the same page, lawyers, courts, and insurance companies were not needed as much to police the doctor-patient relationship. Once upon a time, malpractice and maloccurrence were two different phenomena that were treated differently by a more tolerant and more understanding society.

With all due respect to the legal profession, I still maintain that a doctor's office should be the first place a patient goes to express concern about the health care they have received. I also maintain that physicians should encourage dialogue with their patients and discuss problems in an honest and open manner.

I know two orthopedic surgeons who would agree with this advice. If given the chance to look through the perfectly implanted lens of the retrospectoscope, I'm sure that there's at least one ophthalmologist who would also agree.

April, 1996

LOSING MY MARBLES

Midway through his fifth decade on this mortal coil, an insightful gentleman decided to subject his life to statistical analysis. Considering that his favorite day of the week was Saturday, that there were 52 Saturdays in a year, and that the life expectancy of his generation was 75 years, he reasoned that he could expect to enjoy 3900 Saturdays in his lifetime.

Taking into account his age, the statistician calculated that he had already lived through 2900 Saturdays. This, of course, led to the sobering realization that there might only be an additional 1000 Saturdays left in his entire life.

Thinking about the previous Saturdays that had been wasted and importance of each remaining Saturday, the gentleman went to a toy store and bought 1000 marbles. Placing them in a glass container, he immediately began the ritual of removing one marble each Saturday as a reminder of the short amount of time he had left on this earth.

For nearly two decades, the gentleman watched his supply of marbles dwindle, one at a time, until the day finally came when he removed the final marble from its container. He did so with the satisfaction that his ritual had taught him to respect life and time, and to glean the most out of each passing day.

For the past few years, he has been celebrating each new day as a bonus and refusing to allow any day to end before it has been thoroughly lived and appreciated. He may have lost his marbles, but in doing so, he learned one of life's most important lessons.

There are many who believe that we are all born with our own personalized container of marbles. We gradually lose our marbles until our individual supplies have been depleted and our lives end.

I have been losing my marbles for quite some time—and so have you. Fortunately, the only important marbles are the ones we still have left.

If we really are concerned physicians and thinking individuals, we must ask ourselves how we can best serve our patients and profession before we completely lose our marbles. We must ask ourselves how we can allow the greatest health care delivery system in the history of mankind to be used to its fullest potential.

Today, millions of Americans are unable to afford health care. Millions more must choose between buying prescription drugs or food.

While managed care executives sit in their luxurious offices pondering their portfolios, untold numbers of competent physicians struggle to keep their bills paid and offices open. As many of these physicians read the want ads in hopes of brighter days for themselves and their families, corporate moguls and legislators plan the next move in the on-going socialization of American medicine.

As physicians, it is our responsibility to ready our profession for future generations of healers as well as the masses who will come under their care. As human beings, it is our responsibility to combat the injustices currently depriving millions of their right to be healthy.

For every loss, there is a corresponding gain. If we must lose our marbles, our patients and profession should be the ones who pick up all the marbles we leave behind.

June, 2001

HOUSE CALLS

Back in the 1950's, most of the doctors in our town made house calls. In my neighborhood, which was located on the other side of the proverbial railroad tracks, the kids would rate doctors according to the cars they drove to their patients' homes.

The Cadillac was the gold standard for physicians who drove into our neighborhood to make house calls. Physicians who drove less expensive cars were thought to be inferior caregivers by our neighborhood's pre-pubescent medical review board, while those who occasionally used a house call as a means of showcasing a vehicle, which was slightly more foreign, exotic, or expensive, were given considerably higher professional ratings.

Just like the penicillin shots that seemed to be part of the same ritual, house calls have fallen into disuse by the medical profession. In 1988, American physicians made an estimated 1.6 million house calls while only half that number was made in 1996.

There are many reasons why American physicians are making fewer house calls. For starters, the role of the American physician has changed in recent years, and nurses, therapists, and aides have assumed much of the responsibility of the home health care of elderly, disabled, and chronically ill patients.

Additionally, many physicians have been unable to justify making house calls for financial reasons. House calls have traditionally involved poor reimbursement from third-party payers, uncompensated travel expenses, and the potential for lost income incurred by physicians who spend time away from their offices.

Finally, many physicians are afraid to make house calls because of safety concerns. Unsafe neighborhoods, uncertain home situations, and the onus of trying to render competent medical care without the ancillary personnel, diagnostic equipment, and supplies of the medical office have dissuaded many physicians from treating patients in their homes.

Although many physicians have valid reasons for not making house calls, there are many other reasons why physicians should reconsider the practice. The major reason is the current and projected state of health care in America.

By the time America reaches the 21st Century, the number of medical/surgical beds in American hospitals will be reduced to approximately one-third the numbers mandated by the Hill-Burton Act following World War II. With only 1.5 hospital beds available per 1,000 population, physicians will be forced to develop newer ways to treat both acute and chronic illnesses.

Home health nursing services have already started bridging the gap between the medical office and the hospital, but too many of these services operate sub-optimally because they involve physicians in only a peripheral manner. Homebound patients are generally grateful for the care of their nurses, therapists, and aides, but they would also like to see their physician on a regular basis.

Research studies have clearly demonstrated that patients with chronic or terminal illnesses who see a physician regularly survive significantly longer than patients with similar illnesses who do not see a physician on a regular basis. Homebound patients profit greatly from the services provided by home health nursing services, but such services become much more effective when they are coordinated with the home health care of a physician.

For a number of years, patients have been receiving intravenous medications at home, as well as other therapies that were previously unavailable outside the hospital. The administration of such therapies by home health nursing services has clearly demonstrated the safety and efficacy of treating patients at home.

With the number of hospital beds dwindling and the future financing of health care still uncertain, house calls may become necessary if physicians are to provide timely medical care to patients who are too ill to be treated in a medical office but unable to be hospitalized. Home health care will be able to safely, effectively, and economically bridge the gap between the medical office and the hospital—but not without the active participation of physicians.

In many ways, such a scenario would not be the worst thing that could happen to health care in the United States. In truth, most chronically ill patients would probably prefer to receive medical care in their own home instead of a hospital or extended care facility.

With each hospitalization or institutionalization, patients risk unexpected injury, mental status changes, and nosocomial infections. It is obvious that patients who receive home health care generally do so with levels of comfort and safety that hospitalized patients are usually incapable of obtaining.

I have been making house calls for 17 years, and I can honestly say that the practice has been rewarding both professionally and personally. Patients have profited from my house calls, their families have been grateful for my services, and their communities have been given the chance to see the medical profession up close and personal.

Unlike many of the doctors of the 1950's, I still don't make house calls in a Cadillac. Instead, I usually drive to the rural homes and farms of my patients in my red Firebird convertible.

Fortunately, most of the kids in my neighborhood still think I'm cool. That's probably because the rural town's last doctor drove to his house calls on a John Deere tractor!

February, 1998

NO OTHER FOOTSTEPS
TO FOLLOW

A few months ago, a medical journal published an article I wrote about a country doctor who devoted sixty years of his life to the practice of medicine in rural Vermont. I briefly mentioned his family in the article, but I did not mention that a number of his progeny have followed in his footsteps and become distinguished health care professionals.

One of the doctor's sons is a prominent physician and medical educator, as well as a pioneer in the field of interventional radiology. On reading my article about his father, he sent me a thoughtful letter:

"Dear Bernie, I read your recent article. Thanks for your wonderful recollections and tribute to Dad! There are getting to be fewer of us remaining who have seen and understood the evolution and control of the practice of medicine as it transfers from dedicated individuals with a vocation to the multi-billion dollar corporations and the multi-millionaire CEO's and politicians. The personal and professional caring and attitudes in the patient-physician relationship are 'Gone With The Wind,' or going fast. It will be too late when the patients and society begin to realize what they've turned over and lost to the corporations, executives, lawyers, politicians and government officials. When it was 'The Best Of Times,' things may have been expensive, but the patients and the health givers were the producers and beneficiaries. We are all going to learn what 'The Worst Of Times' will bring! I'm not so sure that Dad is turning over in his grave, but when the cold, hard times were hitting at their worst, that was when he (and we) could do our memorable best. Thanks again for your living memory and literary remembrance of Dad's principles for taking care of his patients. As you know, they will survive any peripheral "money-grabbing" onslaughts and will remain at the heart of the doctor-patient relationship."

The physician who wrote these words has seen it all. His professional life has run the gamut from primary care in a rural setting to military medicine to medical education to specialty medicine in one of the world's most renowned cancer treatment centers.

What all this means is that this physician knows from whence he speaks. It also means that his words are credible and especially meaningful.

When he says, "there are getting to be fewer of us remaining who have seen and understood the evolution and control of the practice of medicine as it transfers from dedicated individuals with a vocation to the multi-billion dollar corporations and the multi-millionaire CEO's and politicians," he pretty much sums up our current health care crisis. Very few physicians know what it means to render care to a patient without the intervention of some insurance company, government agency, or other health care manager.

The vast majority of physicians who still remember what it was like to practice medicine under a free enterprise system have already taken an early retirement from the medical profession rather than opting to suffer the slings and arrows of managed care. Combine this with the fact that the multi-billion dollar corporations and multi-millionaire CEO's and politicians of this world couldn't pick a dedicated individual with a vocation out of a one-man lineup, and the stage is conveniently set for the insidious development of socialized medicine in America.

When this physician says, "the personal and professional caring and attitudes in the patient-physician relationship are 'Gone With The Wind,' or going fast," he points out one of the major differences between medicine as it was practiced in his father's day and medicine as it is regrettably practiced with alarming frequency today. The art of practicing medicine was designed to be personal and professional; the health care rationing of managed care has made medicine impersonal and the health care industry's widespread attempts to pawn physician extenders off as physicians have made it decidedly unprofessional.

His prophetic statement that "it will be too late when the patients and society begin to realize what they've turned over and lost to the corporations, executives, lawyers, politicians and government officials," points out another major difference between his father's medicine and ours. Once upon a time, medicine was practiced by physicians—and only physicians; today, physicians are thought of as mere automatons that carry out the health care mandates of a modern-day power elite.

His admonition that "we are all going to learn what 'The Worst Of Times' will bring," is sobering. Fortunately, it is tempered by the hope that his father's principles "......will survive any peripheral 'money-grabbing' onslaughts and will remain at the heart of the doctor-patient relationship."

Managed care, or socialized medicine as it is called elsewhere, is giving the American medical profession a sneak preview of "The Worst Of Times." Hopefully, the American medical profession will convene in the lobby during the intermission, and somewhere between the popcorn and the chocolate-covered raisins, realize that medicine is too steeped in principles to succumb to the "money-grabbing onslaughts" of the managed care profiteers.

The physician who wrote this letter has a number of children who are also physicians. His children were raised on stories of their grandfather's medical heroics in rural Vermont, and as they listened to the many legends, they watched their own father travel through the most critical metamorphosis in the history of medicine.

Like their father and grand-father, they have each tried to preserve medicine's guiding principles. Avoiding many of medicine's bureaucratic entanglements, they have sponsored free clinics for the poor, and drawing richly from their medical heritage, they have served as voices of reason within their medical communities.

These young physicians are following in the footsteps of their father as well as those of their grand-father. As a result, medicine's time-honored tradition continues to survive.

In the near future, many of us will also have children and grandchildren who are blessed with the same vocation that brought each of us into the medical profession. But what will be our legacy to these children?

Will our legacy be a profession that provides abundant freedom and rich tradition? Or will it be a profession that offers little more than thinly-veiled servitude?

The direction in which each of us steers the medical profession today will help create our children's legacy as well as the legacy of our patients' children tomorrow. This should provide every physician with more than enough incentive to regain control of our profession and preserve its rich heritage for a group of dedicated individuals who will one day have no other footsteps to follow but ours.

March, 1996

THE IMPORTANCE OF SCREENING MAMMOGRAPHY

Fear was apparent in the face of Mary's 10 year-old daughter. "Mommy, do you have cancer?" she asked.

Realizing that her daughter had been recently traumatized by the death of a 40 year-old teacher with breast cancer, Mary chose her words carefully. "Mommy has a breast tumor," she answered, "but not all breast tumors are cancer."

Explaining to her daughter that she was about to undergo a surgical procedure that would hopefully cure her disease, Mary assuaged her daughter's fear. When she finished, Mary realized that she had lessened her daughter's trepidation, but in doing so, had only increased her own.

Shortly after her 40th birthday, Mary saw her gynecologist who, following an unremarkable physical examination, recommended a routine mammogram. Assuring her that he was unable to palpate any breast masses, the gynecologist told Mary that a number of recent scientific studies had suggested that screening mammography was appropriate for women her age.

Following the mammogram, the gynecologist was surprised to learn that the diagnostic study demonstrated a 3.5 centimeter tumor. He found it somewhat difficult explaining to Mary how the mass had been missed on breast examination a few days earlier.

Mary was immediately referred to a surgeon, and a lumpectomy was scheduled. In the two weeks prior to her surgery, Mary experienced a fear of surgery, a fear of what the biopsy might reveal, and a fear of what might happen to her young family if a worse case scenario resulted.

During that period of time, Mary thought about a significant number of other 40 year-old women in her neighborhood who had developed breast cancer or other breast diseases. She also remembered meeting another young woman who, following bilateral radical mastectomies, chemotherapy, radiation therapy, and multiple trips abroad to obtain various miracle cures, succumbed to her illness at the age of 35.

For Mary, a few weeks seemed like an eternity. The question, "Mommy, do you have cancer?" continually ran through her mind.

The medical community is currently renewing debate on whether women between the ages of 40 and 49 should be offered screening mammography. At the present time, various medical societies and research groups are recommending mammograms for women in this age group while other groups of physicians are deeming such routine testing unnecessary.

As a result of this divided opinion, many health insurers, managed care organizations, and government-sponsored health insurance programs are refusing to alter their stance on not paying for screening mammography in women between the ages of 40 and 49. Citing such mammography as medically unnecessary for women in this age group, the health insurance industry is conveniently disregarding the ominous fact that over 30,000 women in their forties are diagnosed with breast cancer each year in the United States.

Significantly, breast cancer is the leading cause of death in women between the ages of 40 and 49. What's more, recent studies suggest that breast cancer mortality can be dramatically reduced in women who begin screening mammography in their forties.

Two recent multi-year, multi-center studies performed in Sweden reported 33% and 44% reductions in breast cancer mortality in women who began screening mammography between the ages of 40 and 49. Even though other recent studies have only demonstrated one-half of the percentage reductions in breast cancer mortality reported in the Swedish studies, it remains incontrovertible that screening mammography begun by women in their forties can dramatically reduce breast cancer mortality by affording earlier breast cancer detection and treatment.

In the past, screening mammography was usually reserved for forty-ish women who possessed any of a number of breast cancer risk factors. These risk factors have been generally thought to include: reproductive factors, such as early menarche, late first birth, nulliparity, late menopause, or a history of not breast-feeding; individual and genetic factors, such as a family history of breast cancer, the presence of benign breast disease, increasing age, tall stature, or increased bone density; environmental factors, such as the use of oral contraceptives, estrogen replacement therapy, alcohol use, exposure to radiation, and exposure to pesticides; and lifestyle factors, such as lack of exercise, obesity, and diets high in calories and saturated fats but low in fruits, vegetables, and fiber.

Unfortunately, more than 25% of women with breast cancer have no known risk factors for the disease. Consequently, in the 40 to 49 year old age group, over 7,500 women without known risk factors can be expected to develop breast cancer each year in the United States.

This, of course, translates into thousands of 40 to 49 year old American women who are currently unaware that they have breast cancer. Such lack of awareness, as well its devastating consequences, would be obviated if screening mammography for women in their forties was encouraged by physicians, endorsed by government, and reimbursed by the health insurance industry.

There are those who continue to argue that self-examination and physical examination by a trained health care professional are adequate to detect the vast majority of breast tumors. These same individuals also argue that screening mammography is an expensive and unnecessary study for most 40 to 49 year old women.

A recent study of thousands of Chinese women clearly demonstrated that breast self-examination is generally unreliable. A recent breast exam by an experienced, board-certified gynecologist clearly demonstrated to Mary that even highly trained health care professionals can miss large breast tumors on close physical examination.

Considering that over 30,000 women in their forties are diagnosed with breast cancer each year in the United States, screening mammography must be made more readily available to women between the ages of 40 and 49. Considering that over 25% of women with breast cancer have no known risk factors for the disease, screening mammography must be made more readily available to all women in this age group.

What's more, physicians must be allowed to recommend screening mammography to 40 year-old women without fear of reprisals by managed care organizations or fear of interference by health insurers. To this end, those currently holding medicine's purse strings must realize that screening mammography and early therapeutic intervention will ultimately prove much less costly than delayed intervention and the protracted treatment of breast cancer's many horrid complications.

By the way, I was just informed that Mary's breast tumor was benign. Mary will be glad to hear the good news, as will her husband and a cute little 10 year-old who can finally be told that mommy doesn't have cancer.

April, 1997

INTERNISTS

W hen I opened my medical practice sixteen years ago, one of my first patients was a teenage boy who experienced life-threatening laryngospasm following minor trauma to the neck. During the boy's brief hospitalization, I discovered that his laryngospasm was a manifestation of underlying angioneurotic edema.

A few weeks later, the boy's mother called to inform me that she was taking her son to another physician for a second opinion. When I inquired why, she told me that one of her neighbors told her I was an internist.

When I acknowledged that I was an internist, the woman informed me she was concerned because an internist was someone who had just graduated from medical school and was still learning how to become a doctor! Realizing any further rebuttal on my part was futile, I encouraged the woman to get her second opinion.

A few days later, the woman called again to thank me for handling her son's emergency, and to express her renewed faith in my ability to practice medicine. A second opinion by an eighty-five year old general practitioner in a neighboring town somehow convinced her that her son did have angioneurotic edema, and that I was qualified to make the diagnosis and treat the condition.

In recent weeks, the medical literature has been abuzz with stories concerning this animal we fondly refer to as an internist. A number of articles have questioned the appropriateness of the term, internist, while other articles have attempted to reestablish the role of the internist in contemporary medicine.

To be sure, the term, internist, can be a confusing one. Although an internist is a highly trained physician who specializes in internal medicine, the designation can be easily confused with the term, intern, a fledgling physician in his or her first year of post-graduate medical education.

What's more, an internist can also be misunderstood as a physician who specializes in gynecological disorders. This, of course, is based on the misconception that "internals," a slang expression for pelvic examinations, are performed, primarily but not exclusively, by internists.

So, if the name, internist, is becoming too cumbersome, what should those of us who practice internal medicine be called? In recognition of the approaching 21st century, perhaps we should adopt a high tech name, like Human Systems Analysts.

Or as a tribute to managed care and its attempts to turn physicians into robots, maybe we should call ourselves Diagnosticons. Or how about Organologists, a term both musical and transcendental!

Appellations notwithstanding, there also appears to be continued controversy over the exact position of the internist on Medicine's totem pole. Specifically, many are questioning if an internist is a medical specialist or a primary care physician.

Historically, internal medicine was created as a medical specialty. Internists were highly trained as medical consultants who could assist primary care physicians, as well as surgeons, in the diagnosis and treatment of medical illnesses.

With time, medical sub-specialists took over many of the responsibilities of the internist, forcing internal medicine specialists to become generalists who spent a greater amount of their professional time in the primary care realm. With the advent of socialized medicine in America, the emphasis in medical care shifted from diagnosis and treatment to prevention, and internists and sub-specialists alike found themselves providing increasingly greater amounts of primary care.

Even though internists go through much more demanding residency training than family practitioners, and even though it is much more difficult to become board certified in internal medicine than it is in family practice, internists and family practitioners are currently being recognized by the federal government and the insurance industry as primary care providers. This trend is reflected in the similar levels of reimbursement internists and family practitioners currently receive from government-sponsored insurance programs.

The power elite that determines Medicine's course have long since decided that American Medicine should be socialized and of a primary care orientation. Hence, the trend to lure an increasingly greater number of medical students into primary care and away from the medical and surgical sub-specialties through manipulation of medical school admissions policies, scholarship and loan distribution, and residency program funding.

Even though internists have been driven deeper into the primary care sector, we still have the distinction of being the only physicians who, by virtue of our intensive training, can bridge the widening chasm between primary care and specialty medicine. Ergo, we, as internists, can still claim the distinction of being both specialists and primary care providers.

All this, of course, would be much more meaningful if we could come up with a better name for ourselves. How about the ***Wakan Wikasa***, which is Native American for "he who everyone turns to when no one else can figure out what's causing the fever?"

February, 1997

HOW TO OBTAIN FREE PRESCRIPTION DRUGS

E ach month, millions of low- to middle-income Americans with chronic illnesses struggle with the prospect of having to pay for their next supply of prescription drugs. Many of these patients can only pay for the medications required to maintain their health by depriving themselves of food or other necessities of life.

These patients have fallen between the cracks of the most advanced health care delivery system in the history of mankind. They make too much money to qualify for Medicaid or other government-sponsored programs that provide prescription drugs, but not enough money to afford health insurance that offers drug coverage, or to pay for medications out-of-pocket without incurring some degree of financial hardship.

Regrettably, most of these Americans, and too many of their physicians, are unaware of the patient assistance programs that are sponsored by most drug manufacturers in the United States. These programs exist to provide free medications to those patients who do not receive drugs through a government-sponsored or third party insurance program and whose financial condition prohibits the purchase of medications used to treat chronic illnesses.

For the record, each drug manufacturer sponsors its own patient assistance program with its own set of participation criteria, but not many of these programs are well publicized. In the past, most physicians have interceded for needy patients and procured drug samples from company representatives or drug vouchers from the companies themselves, but very few physicians have been able to supply their financially-challenged patients with the majority of medications these patients require on a continuing basis.

Five years ago, a group of volunteers saw the need for an agency that could match the specific drug requirements of needy patients with the availability of such medications through the patient assistance programs of the drug manufacturers, and facilitate the delivery of multiple free medications to such patients in an expeditious manner. Their vision has grown into a national organization known as *The Medicine Program*.

Today, *The Medicine Program* attempts to provide free prescription drugs to not only low-income patients who do not qualify for government assistance, do not have insurance coverage for prescription drugs, and cannot afford to buy such medications, but also to middle-income patients who require expensive drugs for the treatment of such conditions as cancer, AIDS, or organ transplant rejection. The majority of *The Medicine Program's* clients are retired, disabled, or in a class of patients whose families incomes range from below the current poverty level to $50,000 yearly.

To take advantage of the organization's benefits, a patient first requests an application from *The Medicine Program* at P.O. Box 515, Doniphan, Missouri 63935-0515, or at their internet site, www.the medicineprogram.com. After listing their name, address, phone number, current prescription drugs, and name and address of their physician, the patient returns the application with a one-time payment of $5 for each prescription drug requested.

After the application is processed, the patient receives a packet from *The Medicine Program* that contains request forms from the manufacturers of the various drugs the patient needs. Most of these forms are straightforward, request a limited amount of financial and family information, and can usually be completed, without assistance, by most senior citizens in 10 to 15 minutes.

These forms allow patients to request multiple drugs that are manufactured by the same company. What's more, they offer the name-brand drugs of the manufacturers rather than generics.

Most of these request forms require a physician's signature that attests to the medical condition and financial need of the patient, and prescriptions for the drugs being requested. Once the forms are completed and the patient has kept copies with which to request future prescription refills, the forms are mailed or faxed from the physician's office to the drug companies.

If approved, the drug companies send a free supply of the medications to the patient's physician within two to three weeks. Although most companies send a three-month supply of their drugs, companies can send a supply lasting from two to twelve months or a voucher that can be redeemed by the patient at most pharmacies.

Each drug company has its own set of patient assistance criteria and each company is responsible for approving the requests for its own drugs. Therefore, a patient who requests a number of different prescription drugs through *The Medicine Program* may only qualify for and receive drugs from a percentage of the companies.

Patients of all ages are entitled to the potential benefits of *The Medicine Program,* and anyone can apply for assistance in obtaining most commonly used prescription drugs. If a patient is determined ineligible to receive free drugs and receives no free drugs through the *The Medicine Program*, he or she is entitled to a full refund of the processing fee which was sent with the initial application.

The Medicine Program is a private company that currently employs ten workers and solicits the help of volunteers. It has never applied for a non-profit tax status, receives no outside funding, and finances its entire operation from the $5 application fees it receives.

Endorsed by a growing number of government and social services programs nationwide, *The Medicine Program* has been used by the State of Illinois human services offices for the past year. *The Medicine Program* currently receives between 1200-1500 applications weekly, and refunds approximately 9% of application fees to patients who do not qualify for drug assistance.

In essence, *The Medicine Program* serves as an agent who matches the prescription drug needs of patients with the available patient assistance programs of drug manufacturers. It is true that patients or their physicians could contact each of the individual drug manufacturers themselves and request application forms for the individual patient assistance programs, but the modest, one-time fee *The Medicine Program* charges for these services seems like a small price to pay for the surprising amount of time, effort, and red tape involved in successfully obtaining free prescription drugs.

I accidentally discovered *The Medicine Program* a few months ago while perusing the newsletter of a state agency that provides social services to the elderly. After interviewing the organization's founder, manager, and one if its workers, I became convinced that *The Medicine Program* is user-friendly, dedicated to its mission, and readily available to answer the questions of patients and physicians.

After interviewing a number of patients who have taken advantage of *The Medicine Program,* I was happy to discover that the program really works. These patients have been receiving free name-brand drugs on a regular basis for prolonged periods of time.

The Medicine Program is no panacea, but for now, it does appear to be one solution to a problem currently confronting a staggering number of Americans who require medications they can't afford. Americans with chronic illnesses and limited financial resources should never have to choose between food and pills, and *The Medicine Program* appears to be one way to obviate such a difficult choice.

July, 2000

SEPTEMBER 11, 2001

Like many other Americans, his outward appearance was deceptive. Slight of build and mild of demeanor, his body never gave any indication that it was housing the soul of a warrior.

Many years ago, he helped America survive the horror that was World War II. From the day he removed his military uniform for the final time, he walked through the country he defended with a pride that only a warrior could begin to understand.

On September 10th, I saw this real-life hero in my office, and heard him say that he never felt better. A few days later, I found myself consoling his wife and trying to convince her that it was a blessing for her 80 year-old husband to have died in his sleep.

He mowed the lawn his final day on earth with an ease and vigor he hadn't displayed in quite some time. Later that evening, he appeared to be dreaming, as if to be engaged in combat, before a final gasp led to a period of sustained silence.

Like most Americans, he sat in front of a television set on September 11th and witnessed the terroristic destruction of the World Trade Center and attack of the Pentagon. Like most warriors, he remained silent, but was unable to conceal the unadulterated anger that coursed throughout his entire body.

CNN didn't list him as one of the casualties of the September 11th attack or televise his funeral. Nevertheless, I'm sure that the tragic events of that day contributed to his death.

Some day, researchers will investigate how many heroes of American wars past died unexpectedly in the days immediately following the terrorism of September 11th. They will tabulate the number of deaths caused by heart attacks, strokes, or other forms of sudden death, and

probably conclude that the stress of witnessing our American home-
land being attacked was contributory.

Other future researches are also inevitable. These are destined to
focus on the vast array of medical and psychological problems acquired
by the survivors of the terroristic attacks on America, as well as the
countless heroes who came to their immediate aid.

Still other studies will focus on the deleterious effects of September
11th on the families and friends of attack victims and rescuers alike.
Many Americans were killed or injured because of terrorism on September 11th, but many others succumbed to aftermath.

In the hours immediately following the terroristic attacks, over
7,000 American physicians volunteered to assist in the delivery of
emergency medical care to the New York City area alone. Thousands
of other physicians volunteered to help in our nation's capitol or anywhere else they were needed.

Many other physicians prepared to have their military reserve status
upgraded to active duty. Still other physicians prepared to pick up the
slack and handle the inevitable increase in health problems about to
befall a country destined for war.

On September 11th, America's physicians were not thinking about
malpractice cases or managed care, and injured Americans were not
complaining about the cost of health insurance or a doctor surplus.
Instead, physicians were asking each other what we could do to protect
and serve the country we love, and Americans were thanking God for
their immediate access to competent medical care.

Throughout history, the United States has suffered many crises that
could not have been resolved without the help of its physicians. History can be expected to repeat itself and America's physicians stand
prepared to ensure the health and well-being of the greatest nation on
earth.

September, 2001

SANTA CLAUS

For longer than anyone could remember, he was the rural community's pharmacist. A skilled compounder of prescriptions, he was conversant in chocolates, greeting cards, and how to obviate a trip to the doctor's office by using an over-the-counter remedy.

A devoted family man, he was involved in many civic and church activities. Most have forgotten all the roles he once played in the community, but no one will ever forget that he was Santa Claus.

Every Christmas Eve, the town's children would flock to the church hall to sit on his lap and exchange wish lists for candy canes. Every year, at least one imp would tug on his fake beard and publicly proclaim, "You ain't Santa Claus—you're Buzz from the drug store!"

Like Clark Kent and Don Diego de la Vega, he allowed his everyday existence to mesh with that of his alter ego. His name was Buzz, and he worked in a drug store—but he was also Santa Claus.

Buzz was a wise old elf who realized that it took more than one day a year to complete Santa's work. Accordingly, he was always available to provide doctors with medications for late night or week-end emergencies, dispense free pharmacology lessons with the prescriptions he filled, and even refer patients to doctors who stocked samples of medications the patients needed but couldn't afford.

He also realized that Santa's work was too much for any one man and that a number of chronic illnesses would ultimately force him to relinquish Santa's chair. With this in mind, he taught others his skills to ensure that the sick would always have cures, the needy would always have friends, and children of all ages would always have a Santa Claus.

Today, pharmacists he helped train are continuing his charitable practices, corpulent men with real white beards are competing for the chance to carry on holiday traditions he helped establish, and others who remember his gentle kindness are extending the spirit of giving from a season to a lifetime. Buzz preached the gospel according to Saint Nick and his ability to practice what he preached attracted many future Santas.

For too many Americans, Christmas will not arrive soon enough this year. For others, the day, season, and spirit may not come at all.

Tragedy came to America on September 11, 2001, but it has given no indication that it plans to leave any time soon. Until it decides to leave, our American way of life will be disrupted.

There are many American children and adults who are currently frightened, confused, and worried. They need the grace of God and strength of all that is symbolized by our flag, but they also need kindness, comfort, and support.

When I think of kindness, the image of Santa Claus immediately comes to mind. When I think of Santa, I think of Buzz—my colleague, patient, and friend for more than 20 years.

Buzz died a few days ago, but before he did, he willed the title of Santa Claus to anyone who understood that one of life's greatest gifts was a willingness to give. He died with the hope that each of us would allow Santa Claus to emerge from our personalities and contribute an added measure of kindness to our troubled world.

When the **_Book of Medicine_** is finally completed, some physicians will be remembered as Surgeon General, some as President of the American Medical Association, and some as Director of the Centers for Disease Control. If there is a line in the book for me, I'd like to be remembered as a country doctor who once took care of Santa Claus.

November, 2001

FINAL THOUGHTS

I just returned from the hospital where I admitted my patient, Pete, yesterday. He developed a severe case of bronchitis, and his coughing, wheezing, and shortness of breath became too much to handle on an out-patient basis.

He's doing a lot better today. In fact, doing better is what Pete has been all about for the past few years.

When you consider that the man has had 5 heart attacks, 2 open-heart surgeries, and just about every other problem discussed in any medical textbook, saying that Pete is doing better is saying an awful lot. Pete is a prime example of what modern medicine has been able to accomplish in the past 20 years.

Pete is also a prime example of a human being whose pain and suffering have frequently been caused by factors unrelated to poor health. He typifies the many Americans who have fallen between the cracks of the most sophisticated health care delivery system in the history of the world.

I am extremely proud of all I have been able to do medically for Pete as his doctor. I am just as proud of all I have been able to do to ease the pain and suffering Pete has experienced as an incredibly-ill American who has been unable to afford the many medications he requires to sustain his health and very existence.

When I first wrote about Pete and his wife, Jan, in my essay, **Choices**, I was unaware of the information I presented in my later essay, **How To Obtain Free Prescription Drugs**. Specifically, I was unaware of any programs that were providing free prescription drugs for needy patients.

When I finally became aware of **The Medicine Program** a few years later, I helped Pete enroll. Since that time, he has been obtaining his prescription drugs free of charge.

Pete's multiple medical conditions, including diabetes mellitus, hypertension, and congestive heart failure, require many different medications. By showing him how to obtain these medications without cost, I have saved him thousands of dollars yearly, and allowed him and his wife to lead more comfortable and less stressful lives.

Practicing medicine from the heart requires a willingness to be a person's friend as well as that person's doctor. It requires a willingness to go the extra step and do things for people that transcend the traditional boundaries of the doctor-patient relationship.

My patients, Sara and Ray, who I wrote about in **The Art of Medicine**, died a few years ago. I considered both of them my friends as well as patients, and during their many severe illnesses, they welcomed my friendship as much as my medical care.

A number of other patients who I have written about in this book are also deceased, but most of the patients you have met in the preceding pages, are alive and well. They continue to provide me with more real-life experiences than any author could ever write about in one lifetime.

I just received another card from Jerry and his wife, reminding me that it has been 19 years since I helped him survive his 2 cardiac arrests. He's 75 years-old now, and although he and his wife don't travel as much as they used to, they continue to enjoy their lives and remain grateful for the help I once provided.

The 3 kids who learned how to hit a baseball on **A Bare Patch Of Ground** are also doing very well. Chris is now a third-year medical student, Ali is a first-year medical student, and Matt is a second-year pre-med student.

Their mother, and my wife of 28 years, is also doing well. The practice of medicine has cost too many physicians their marriages and families, but nowhere is it written that successful family lives and successful careers have to be mutually exclusive.

My wife and 3 children have always been my top priority in life. My devotion to my family has made me a better person which, in turn, has made me a better doctor.

Many of the health care issues discussed in this book are still unresolved. Technologically, the medical profession continues to advance, while our nation's ability to deliver health care to every American in a competent, timely, and affordable manner continues to lag far behind our technological achievements, and continues to be stifled by forces outside the medical profession.

You and I still have a lot to discuss about health care in America. Hopefully, we can continue our discussion in my next book, ***MEDICINE BETWEEN THE LINES***.

In the meantime, I have patients to see, and miles to go before I can record today's experiences for posterity. I don't know what today will bring, but I do know that I have been blessed with one more day to practice Medicine—from the heart.

August, 2002

0-595-24502-1